# The
# RealAge®
# *Workout*

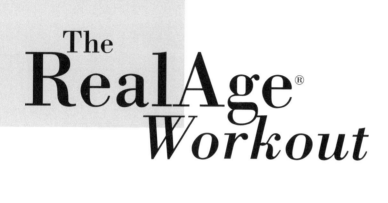
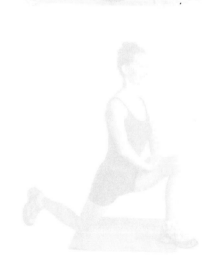

## Also by Michael F. Roizen, M.D.

*YOU: The Owner's Manual* (with Mehmet C. Oz, M.D.)

*YOU: The Smart Patient* (with Mehmet C. Oz, M.D.)

*The RealAge® Makeover*

*RealAge®: Are You As Young As You Can Be?*
    (with Elizabeth Anne Stephenson)

*The RealAge® Diet: Make Yourself Younger with What You Eat*
    (with John La Puma, M.D.)

*Cooking the RealAge® Way* (with John La Puma, M.D.)

# The RealAge® Workout

## Workout

MAXIMUM HEALTH, MINIMUM WORK

Michael F. Roizen, M.D.
Tracy Hafen, M.S.

With Lawrence A. Armour

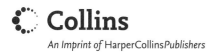

**Collins**

*An Imprint of HarperCollinsPublishers*

This book is intended to be informational and should not be considered a substitute for advice from a medical professional, whom the reader should consult before beginning any diet or exercise regimen, and before taking any dietary supplements or other medications. The authors and the publisher expressly disclaim responsibility for any adverse effects arising from the use or application of the information contained in this book.

All case studies portrayed in this book are based on real people. Some details insignificant to the examples in this book have been changed to protect the identities of the individuals. In some cases, two or more similar stories have been combined into one story. Only references to Tracy and me remain clearly identifiable. Any other likenesses are purely coincidental.

In certain instances, I have listed products by their brand names—for example, specific exercise machines—since that is how they are commonly known. I have occasionally also included names of companies and products, if I thought that mentioning the name provided relevant information for the reader. To my knowledge, I have no connections to any of the companies or brand-name products listed in this book, with the exception of RealAge, Inc., the company which I helped found for the express purpose of developing the RealAge scientific evidence and computer program, and other RealAge programs. RealAge and Age Reduction are trademarks and service marks of RealAge, Inc. RealAge, Inc. currently directs the RealAge Web site (www.RealAge.com).

### Note About the Format of the Book

We've written this book in the first person to make it easier to read. But everywhere you see an "I," you can assume a "we."

HarperCollins books may be purchased for educational, business, or sales promotional use. For information, please write: Special Markets Department, HarperCollins Publishers, 10 East 53rd Street, New York, NY 10022.

FIRST EDITION

*Designed by Jaime Putorti*

All photographs by Greg Gillis

Library of Congress Cataloging-in-Publication Data has been applied for.

ISBN-10: 0-06-000937-3
ISBN-13: 978-0-06-000937-3

06   07   08   09   10   WBC/QW   10   9   8   7   6   5   4   3   2   1

All of my patients knew they should exercise before they saw me—yet less than 5 percent knew what that meant or how little they needed to do for maximum health benefits. I wrote this book to end that confusion—to tell you what is known about the types and amounts of exercise you need to maximally slow your rate of aging. This book is dedicated to all those patients who teach me and who teach other health professionals to be better than we are.

# Contents

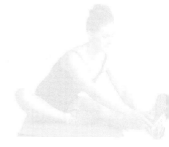

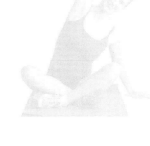

# Acknowledgments

Anesthesia and internal medicine, the two specialties I am boarded in and practice, interface substantially in the preoperative care of patients. It is in that sphere where I try to encourage patients to adopt healthier behaviors in the one to eight weeks prior to surgery. That process enables each patient to have the greatest chance of a full functional recovery and a higher quality of life after surgery. I need to acknowledge my closest mentors in anesthesia and internal medicine, Bill Hamilton and Ken Melmon, who encouraged this work. Without them, a preoperative clinic founded on the principle that patients can become healthier prior to surgery and procedures, and thereby improve their life and safety, would never have been conceived, let alone flourish.

It was in these attempts that the concept of RealAge® was born—to inform patients of just how much control everyone had over his or her genes (that's the science) and how easy it was to make important differences in outcome. And to motivate them to change. I was privileged to develop that data in weekly sessions with Keith Roach, informed by the direct work of the RealAge Scientific Advisory Board of Axel Goetz, Tate Erlinger, and Harriet Imrey. As we read the works of Steven Blair, Ralph Paffenbarger, and others about what physical activities it takes to attain optimal health, we were struck that so many books, fitness gurus, trainers, and even medical articles preached behaviors not supported by science. Then I met Tracy Hafen, and as we developed a program grounded in these scientific principles that tried to reverse aging, and tested it on patients, we began to find remarkable results—people looked, felt, and became younger. And when the *RealAge* books and RealAge Web site began to spread this motivating metric and these scientific principles, we were deluged by a hundred and fifty thank-you e-mails a day.

These e-mail writers are the real people to whom an acknowledgment is owed— their thank-you notes told the easiest method to adopt this science. Yes, we knew the exercises to keep you younger, but it was the e-mails that taught us how individuals who were just plain typical people, and not the athletic superheroes required by many bodybuilding books, could adopt these activities. Easily. We tested it on our patients— and low and behold, it worked. So the literally tens of thousands of e-mail writers are the ones who really deserve credit for this program.

Many colleagues in other specialties at the Cleveland Clinic provided content and deserve gratitude, especially my administrative associate Beth Grubb; the very supportive public-affairs group at the Clinic including Jim Blazar, Eileen Sheil, and Mary Claire Burick taught me to stay on message. And a special thanks goes to Jennifer Perciballi of RealAge, Myrna Pudersen and Joan McGrath, and many others who taught me much about how to present ideas. I must also thank Toby Cosgrove, Joe Hahn, Mike O'Boyle, Bob Llamas, and Mike O'Donnell, who make wellness a daily priority at the Cleveland Clinic, and Dean Harrison, who makes it a priority at Northwestern Memorial Hospital.

I am grateful to the many, many other people who contributed to this book. Some deserve a very specific thank you: Candice Fuhrman for making it happen—she has been a consistent and constant partner. Nothing in the series of books written with my input that aim to change the health of the nation would have happened without her. Also I would like to thank Larry Armour for helping with the editing and organization of the book, and encouraging it; Elsa Dixon, who rewrote and edited many editions of each chapter; Elizabeth Stephenson, my partner in the first *RealAge* book, who taught me that writing books could be fun; Sukie Miller, whose passion for the project proved to be the consistent encouragement needed to start the *RealAge* and *YOU* sequence of books; Anita Shreve for saying this *RealAge* book was possible and that the chapters were just what she wanted to read; the many gerontologists and internists who read sections of the book for accuracy; Steven Blair, Ralph Paffenbarger, Jack Rowe, Jeremiah Stamler, Linda Fried, and the many investigators of the Iowa Women's Health Study, the Nurses' Health Study, and the Physicians' Health Study, for invaluable research and advice that improved the science in this book; others on the RealAge Scientific Advisory Board who helped analyze the research, especially Keith Roach, a consistent partner in this work since 1994; those on the RealAge team who helped validate and verify the content, including Shelly Bowen; Anne-Marie Prince for doing so much so well, and for doing it so calmly in the midst of a constant storm; Sally Kwa, Arline McDonald, Linda Van Horne, Mark Rudberg, and Mike Parzen for their roles as scientific partners in evaluating the data and scientific content of RealAge; Sidney Unobskey and Martin Rom, who inspired the process and named it; Charlie Silver, who funded the research and assembled the innovative RealAge team that continually evaluates and updates RealAge and its Web site. I owe a special gratitude to Kathryn Huck-Seymour, who repeatedly told me how to improve each chapter; she made each chapter better, and not just a little, and not just once. I also owe a special thanks to Mehmet C. Oz, my partner in the *YOU* books, who unselfishly gave of time and who said this book was needed, and encouraged it and made it better.

I want to acknowledge three special people as well: Diane Reverand stated, "Not to worry about offending medical colleagues—as long as the science was solid, they would understand you were trying to motivate readers to understand they could control their own health and were responsible for doing so and for enjoying the extra energy and vitality"; Kandi Amelon, who pushed us to get better; and of course Tracy Hafen.

No one deserves more thanks for persistence or creativity than Tracy, my partner in this book, who with infinite patience worked with me and our patients to improve their lives. And after that, and while caring for six children, still found time to write the book and keep making it better.

I also want to thank Nancy for her constant love and support. Our children, Jeffrey and Jennifer, read and helped make the series of *RealAge* books better. So did Nancy, who lives the RealAge Workout, and used her expertise in critical reading to make our work better. She proves that even cynics can become believers in the

RealAge Workout and relish the extra vigor and life it gives. She makes my life better daily.

I hope this book will help you progressively adopt physical activity into your life and enjoy Maximum Health with Minimum Work. That would be the best gift any physician could receive.

—Michael F. Roizen, M.D.

A heartfelt thanks goes to those who worked on this book in a tangible way. First, thanks to Steve Tober for volunteering his time as a model for the exercise photos. Steve kept me and the photographer laughing through the entire and rather grueling two days of shooting. Second, Greg Gillis, the photographer, exhibited not only great skill but also great patience in working with us. I also need to thank Greg's colleague, Chris Morris, the photo editor, for the almost countless hours spent in outlining every picture to give each the detail and quality we wanted. Finally, I wish to express my gratitude to Wendy Randall, Elsa Dixon, and Larry Armour for their editing expertise.

My thanks also go out to the many people who helped with this book in a more indirect way. Alexia Koelling, my friend and running partner, heard my barrage of ideas, complaints, and discoveries, and she always kept me running while providing sound insights at the same time. The sportswear companies Hind®, REI®, Adidas®, Road Runner Sports®, and Under Armour® provided valuable information on exercise gear and clothing. I also wish to thank those personal trainers and physical therapists from my past who solidified my belief in the fitness industry: Mark Bayers, Joanna O'Keefe, Sara Blakely, Aimee Barnas, Kirsten Minor, Pam Birnie, Larry Kempton, Holly Smiley, Greg Booth, Sara Madsen, Roberto Pelosi, and Robert Lardner. They always conducted themselves professionally and made the welfare of their clients a top priority.

Perhaps most important to me in this book endeavor have been my long-term clients, some of whom have been with me since I first began working with clients of my own more than ten years ago. They have seen our family through ten years of graduate school and six children, and have been supportive through all of the schedule changes, maternity leaves, periods of neglect and absentmindedness, and all the joys and crises of life. They have truly become my closest friends, and I hope we are all the healthier for it. In particular I wish to thank Lynn Frackman and Tom Meites, Claire Dankoff, Jerome Winer, Marie Krane-Bergman, and Rabbi Arnold Wolf. You all continue to mean much to me.

Of course I need to thank Dr. Roizen. I attended a book talk of his at 57th Street Book in Hyde Park, Chicago. I was impressed by his presentation, and after the book-signing line died down, I handed him a card with my name and number, and explained that I would love to help him with a workout book if he ever chose to write one. He called a few months later, and our collaboration began. His hand in my life has shaped the path my career has taken (and is taking) more than he realizes. And his personal example of hard work, integrity, tireless energy, and love of his field continues to amaze me. I am convinced that the main goal and motive in his work is to improve the lives and health of people everywhere, even if it is one person at a time. I see it drive him, and I appreciate the example.

Lastly, I'm grateful for my husband, Tom, who has actively supported me in this project, not only with his ideas but with his hours of watching the kids so that I could get a little work done. The same could be said for my mother, JoEllen Taylor, who flew out on more than one occasion to give me some concentrated time to work. I also thank my children, Daniel, Chaya, Caleb, Elia, Asher, and Micah, for being the kind of kids who make motherhood the most rewarding job in the world and who give me my greatest reason for keeping as healthy as possible.

—Tracy Hafen, M.S.

# The
# RealAge®
# *Workout*

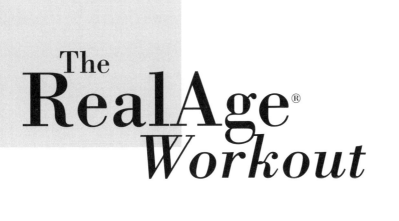

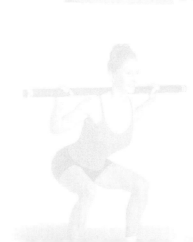

# The RealAge® Promise

## Lazy? No, Just Time-Challenged

"Tell me the truth, Mike. What's the MINIMUM amount of physical activity I must do to produce the MAXIMUM health benefit?" This is a great question I'm often asked by my patients who—busy with careers or family, with little free time to spare—still want to safeguard their health and their futures. Perhaps you have wondered this, too. Well, the answer is now in your hands. Whether you want to regain the vigorous health of your youth, stay feeling as good as you do today in the years to come, or get into even better shape than ever while slowing your rate of aging, *The RealAge® Workout* will show you how.

What is the program based on? The RealAge Scientific Advisory Board has reviewed over 35,000 scientific studies on aging, over 5,000 alone on the effects of exercise on health, and has culled the wheat from the chaff. The kernels have been tested and proven (and reproven time and time again) on my patients, and now I'm going to give them to you. I will help you create a goal of how young you want to be, and design a concrete plan that will help you to achieve your goal.

The wonderful truth is that aging is a process that you can control. There are literally hundreds of steps you can take—things you can do—that will enable you to play golf, relish conversations or crossword puzzles, travel to faraway places, dance the night away, and even climb mountains until near the day you die. That, in a nutshell, is what the RealAge concept is all about.

The RealAge system:

- Allows you to know how old you *really* are—in biological, not chronological, terms. (To determine your RealAge, take the test at www.realage.com.)
- Enables and motivates you to change your RealAge and develop the health profile of someone who is chronologically many years younger. (Today, a 75-year-old man can make his RealAge 27 years younger than his calendar age and a 75-year-old woman can make her RealAge 29 years younger than her calendar age.)
- Views health not as the prevention of disease but as the prevention of aging.
- Is based on scientific data that you can slow the pace of aging and actually reverse it. You can control which of your genes are turned on or off—all genes do is make proteins or regulate other genes, and which of your genes are turned on is in your control.

Research has demonstrated that lifestyle choices and behavior have a far greater impact on longevity and health than heredity. And choosing to be physically active is one of the most important lifestyle choices. Unfortunately, many people think they don't have enough time to devote to exercise to really make a difference. Luckily, they're wrong. I wrote this book because I want you to benefit from what the hundreds of RealAge–Partnership Medicine patients and the millions of RealAge members taught me about the minimum exercise we need to achieve the maximum health benefit. And the good news is small amounts of time can make a huge difference to your health, your well-being, and your RealAge.

Sounds too good to be true, doesn't it? I thought so, too, until I saw the amazing transformations of patients—and some strangers—who followed the RealAge Workout plan, some for only 10 minutes at a time. (Most of the strangers became friends.)

So what is the RealAge Workout, exactly? It's simple—a program broken into four

30-day phases that build one upon the other, slowly getting you to the physical activity that will ensure the optimal level of health for you (with the minimum necessary time commitment). Once you've completed the four 30-day phases, you will be at your best possible level of health facilitated by exercise. You'll feel great and have the energy to do all the things you love and the peace of mind to know you're taking great care of your health. Best of all, the plan is easy and fun.

## Overview of the Plan

- ■ Phase 1 (Days 1–30): Walk 30 minutes every day—either all at once or 10 minutes or more at a time.
- ■ Phase 2 (Days 31–60): Increase your level of activity by adding 7–10 minutes of strength training of your foundation muscles every other day.
- ■ Phase 3 (Days 61–90): Increase your level of activity by adding 8–10 minutes of strength training of your non-foundation muscles★ every other day.
- ■ Phase 4 (Days 91 Onward): Increase your level of activity with 21† minutes of stamina or aerobic exercises, 3 times a week.

Sound simple? It is. But don't let the simplicity of the plan fool you into thinking you can jump a phase, or shorten a phase to 15 days instead of 30. For important scientific and medical reasons, success is more likely if you follow the gradual buildup, order, and time frame of the plan.

For example, even if you're excited to get started and feel you could do more, don't skip Phase 1 to start strength-building exercises right away. Your muscles must undergo two specific changes to regain youth and strength. As your muscle ages, it loses the contractile proteins (that give a muscle strength) and the proteins that make the energy factory of your cells (mitochondrial—these give your muscle stamina). To regain strength, you need to rebuild (or build) contractile proteins; to regain stamina, you need to recondition your mitochondrial functions.

---

★ The differences between foundation and non-foundation muscles are explained in Chapter 3.
† Most ask why 21 and not 20 minutes—wish it were a "round" number. Those are the data: 21 minutes 3 times a week is the minimal time for maximum benefit; since RealAge is data driven, we use the "21" and not "20."

By simply walking, you start doing both. If you walk 30 minutes a day for 30 days, you rebuild enough of the energy factories in your muscles to progress to safely building strength proteins. And you have to rebuild enough strength proteins so your first attempt at resistance exercise will not rip a joint or muscle apart. Therefore, Phase 1 is a necessary step. Best of all, by simply walking for 30 minutes every day, you can make your RealAge younger by 2.2 years.

Resistance exercises, which you do in Phases 2 and 3, build and strengthen muscles and bones, and keep them in top form. It's vital that you build up your foundation muscles first in Phase 2 so that you are strong and steady at your core, and less prone to injury before you start resistance exercises on your non-foundation muscles.

Although strength building by itself contributes just 20 percent to your overall Age Reduction, don't underestimate its value. Strength-building activities boost contractile proteins and energy, lessen stress, and provide an insurance policy for your body by helping prevent injury. Doing strength-building or resistance exercises for 10 minutes a day, 3 times a week, is also one of the best ways to get an immediate energy boost.

Once you've built up your strength and endurance in the first 90 days of the plan, then—and only then—should you begin stamina-building activities (Phase 4). Stamina-building activities raise your heart rate, and are what most people commonly think of as exercise: jogging, biking, swimming, and aerobics. Through vigorous exercise—any physical activity that makes you break a sweat and causes your heart to beat faster—you can make your RealAge 3.7 years younger.

Any exercises that cause you to sweat for 21 minutes have a double benefit: They not only count toward the 63 minutes of stamina exercise per week that produces optimum age reduction (3.7 years younger for this), but they also burn extra calories (an overall physical activity goal) toward the 3,500 calories per week that will make you an additional 3.7 years younger. Calories consumed in all three categories (walking, strength, and stamina) count toward your overall activity goal. And each of these three has a separate and different effect on your rate of aging. None alone will make your RealAge younger by more than 3.7 years, but together they can take a whopping 9.1 years off your biologic clock. Let's have a look at the numbers on the opposite page.

## Table 1.1
## The RealAge Effect of The RealAge Workout Plan*

For Men:
Kilocalories Expended Per Week
(doing all three components gets you to ideal of 3500–6499[†])

| CALENDAR AGE | LESS THAN 500 | 500–2,000 | 2,000–3,500 | 3,500–6,500 | MORE THAN 6,500 |
|---|---|---|---|---|---|
| | | | REALAGE | | |
| 35 | 36.7 | 35 | 33.1 | 31.4 | 32.4 |
| 55 | 57.7 | 55 | 53.3 | 49.6 | 52 |
| 70 | 73.9 | 70 | 69 | 65.2 | 68.7 |

For Women:
Kilocalories Expended Per Week
(doing all three components gets you to ideal of 3500–6499[†])

| CALENDAR AGE | LESS THAN 500 | 500–2,000 | 2,000–3,500 | 3,500–6,500 | MORE THAN 6,500 |
|---|---|---|---|---|---|
| | | | REALAGE | | |
| 35 | 36.7 | 35 | 33.1 | 31.4 | 32.4 |
| 55 | 57.9 | 55 | 52.3 | 48.8 | 51.6 |
| 70 | 74.2 | 70 | 68.3 | 64.6 | 67.1 |

* These benefits or RealAge effects are calculated for the physical activity alone, and exclude the benefits of blood pressure reduction, stress reduction, better blood sugar and blood lipid control, anti-inflammatory effects, etc. So the benefit is really much greater. Further, such calculations assume you do the average amount of every other behavior in the RealAge program—see our Web site www.realage.com or Chapter 2 in *The RealAge Makeover* for a more complete explanation of these calculations and the scientific bases of these calculations.
† Assumes you also do *some* physical activity in daily living besides exercise like making beds or taking out the garbage.

Pretty straightforward, right? But before we start, let's map out the journey you'll be taking. Start with where you are, Point A.

## Where Are You?

To map a journey to a younger you, begin by plotting two important points: Point A, where you are on the fitness map, and Point B, where you want to go. "Easy enough," you say to yourself. "I'm stuck in Portlyland and I'd like to get to Fitsburg." Unfortunately, you'll have to be a little more specific.

A variety of easy tests can tell you how your physical activities have influenced your rate of aging and your current RealAge. These tests will then help you establish your personal goals. We will show you how to take each one, and then—armed with the information they provide—move from Point A, your current location, to Point B, the destination you'd like to reach.

The tests will ascertain:

- Your non-stressed (resting) heart rate.
- Your non-stressed (resting) blood pressure.
- Your exercise capacity.
- Your muscular strength, endurance, and flexibility.
- Your body composition (waist, weight).

You will record the results of these five tests on the progress sheet on page 24. Later, once you're in Phase 4 and doing regular stamina exercise, you will do two more tests to determine:

- Your heart rate at maximum exercise.
- Your heart rate 2 minutes after maximum exercise (2-minute recovery heart rate).

To find your Point A, examine your overall health. You must decide if you should seek advice from your physician before starting. **You definitely need to see a doctor before you do the tests that follow (and before you start your RealAge walking program) if:**

- Your doctor has told you not to walk.
- You have chest pain or heaviness or shortness of breath without doing any activity.
- You are unstable, lose balance easily, or get dizzy when you walk.
- You take medications, especially for blood pressure. (Some medications affect your balance or exercise heart rate and could influence how you walk.)

Most adults do **not** need to talk to a doctor before beginning a walking plan of moderate intensity, but should see one before they start resistance or stamina training. This process can be accomplished by calling your doctor when you first start to walk, because such a preventive visit often takes 30 days to arrange.

## Resting Heart Rate

Most of us have a resting heart rate between 60 and 76 beats per minute. The resting heart rates of very sedentary and unconditioned people (or people with certain diseases) can measure well over 80 beats per minute; on the other end of the spectrum, the rates of highly trained endurance athletes typically range between 35 and 50 beats per minute.

To obtain your resting heart rate:

1. Sit in a comfortable position for at least 10 minutes while listening to music or doing something relaxing. The most accurate readings are those taken first thing in the morning or immediately following a nap while you're still lying down.

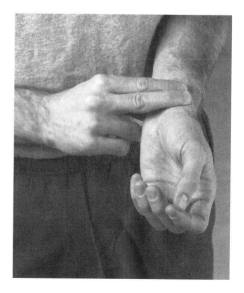

2. Using the tips of your middle and index fingers, find your pulse on the thumb side of your wrist or on the side of your neck.

3. Count the number of beats you feel during a 60-second period. Record this number. It is your resting heart rate. It's a good idea to take the measurements on two separate occasions, perhaps on consecutive days, and then take the average of the two results.

If your resting heart rate is greater than 75 beats per minute your RealAge is older than your calendar age (see Table 1.2 opposite); a resting heart rate greater than 83 indicates a considerably older RealAge; a resting heart rate greater than 92 probably means you should see your physician soon.

If you want a more exact measure of your heart rate, buy a heart rate monitor. This device—generally composed of a monitor watch and a strap that goes around your chest—is available at most sporting goods stores or on the Internet: Just type "sports heart rate monitors" into a search engine. The monitor consists of a sensor that picks up the electrical impulse that is your heartbeat, plus a transmitter that sends the information to the watch. These monitors are accurate, last a long time, and are not terribly costly.

## Blood Pressure

While your resting heart rate has a RealAge effect measured in months, the effect of your blood pressure can be measured in many years.

Why do you feel less energy than you did when you were nine years old? That's easy. As your calendar age gets older, your arteries age. They get harder and are less able to dilate and constrict. That's what high blood pressure—or hypertension, as it's generally called—causes. It makes your arteries harder and robs you of energy because hardened arteries cannot dilate as much, as easily, or—at times—even at all. So you can't get the oxygen-rich blood flowing to the working muscles.

This process is common, but not inevitable. Hardening of the arteries and hypertension do not need to happen. As people following the RealAge workout demonstrate, physical activity actually *reverses* this process.

## What the Numbers Mean

You are probably familiar with having your blood pressure checked. What is being measured is the amount of force your blood is putting on the arteries as it flows through them. For example, 129/86 is the median blood pressure for Americans in their mid- to late-forties and early fifties. The top number in the fraction is the systolic pressure, or the pressure that's exerted on the artery walls when the heart beats. The bottom number, the diastolic pressure, is the pressure exerted on your artery walls when the heart is at rest between beats.

## Table 1.2
## The RealAge Effect of Your Resting Heart Rate*

### For Men:

| CALENDAR AGE | 35–67 | 68–75 | 76–83 | 83–92 | OVER 92 |
|---|---|---|---|---|---|
| | | | REALAGE | | |
| 35 | 33.7 | 34.0 | 36.6 | 37.2 | 38.5 |
| 55 | 53.5 | 53.9 | 56.6 | 57.3 | 58.8 |
| 70 | 68.4 | 68.8 | 71.7 | 72.5 | 74.1 |

YOUR RESTING HEART RATE

### For Women:

| CALENDAR AGE | 35–67 | 68–75 | 76–83 | 83–92 | OVER 92 |
|---|---|---|---|---|---|
| | | | REALAGE | | |
| 35 | 34.6 | 34.7 | 35.6 | 36.2 | 36.6 |
| 55 | 54.5 | 54.6 | 55.6 | 56.2 | 56.7 |
| 70 | 69.5 | 69.6 | 70.7 | 71.2 | 71.8 |

YOUR RESTING HEART RATE

* These benefits or RealAge effects are calculated for this measurement alone. Further, such calculations assume you do the average amount of every other behavior in the RealAge program—see our Web site www.realage.com or Chapter 2 in *The RealAge Makeover* for a more complete explanation of these calculations and the scientific bases of these calculations.

The higher your blood pressure, the more stress you are putting on your heart, and the more nicks, bumps, and potholes you create in your arteries.

Blood pressure is often elevated when you are anxious, upset, or hurried. But every elevation of blood pressure means needless aging. Just being in a doctor's office can raise your blood pressure. If that's the case for you, don't avoid the doc; just find out how to make your blood pressure normal, a task that often involves the types of physical activity found in the RealAge Workout.

## What percent of my friends are likely to have high blood pressure?

Eighty-nine percent of Americans have blood pressure higher than 115/76, the ideal for preventing aging. Nearly a quarter have blood pressure above the American Heart Association's danger zone of 140/90. Even the old standard that many consider ideal—120/80—is too high for optimal health and youth.

Bottom line:

■ Hardening of your arteries does not have to happen.

■ A physical activity program almost always reduces your blood pressure.

■ By keeping your blood pressure at the ideal level of 115/76, you can make your RealAge 6 to 10 years younger than if your blood pressure were at the national median of 129/86.

■ Almost all of us can attain the ideal level of 115/76.

## Body Composition and Size

If their TV set and their refrigerator weren't in two different rooms, some people wouldn't get any exercise at all. If this is true for you, you are going to see and feel a real difference in the shape of your body when you walk regularly. Even if you have never exercised consistently, you can, with the RealAge Workout program, reach the best shape of your life at age 40, 50, 60, or even 70. As a fit 70-year-old, you can literally feel better and be younger than you were as an unfit 45-year-old.

No matter what your size, you should record your starting point. First, weigh yourself on the scale you normally use. Do it first thing in the morning, while naked. Then, set a target or goal. Many people try to achieve the weight they were at age 18 or 21. That's usually unrealistic. I urge my patients to aim for a more attainable target— say, a weight that is 10 to 15 pounds heavier than your weight in high school or college

## Table 1.3

# The RealAge Effect of Combinations of Diastolic and Systolic Blood Pressure Readings

(Find your diastolic blood pressure in the left hand column, then move across the row to find your systolic blood pressure; then move down the column to find the RealAge effect of your blood pressure.)

### For Men:

| DIASTOLIC BLOOD PRESSURE (MM HG) | | SYSTOLIC BLOOD PRESSURE (MM HG) | | | |
|---|---|---|---|---|---|
| LESS THAN 80 | LESS THAN 120 | 120 TO 129 | 130 TO 139 | 140 TO 159 | GREATER THAN 160 |
| CALENDAR AGE | | REALAGE | | | |
| 35 | 30.2 | 32.2 | 33.9 | 35.6 | 40.4 |
| 55 | 47.3 | 50.4 | 53.1 | 58.8 | 62.4 |
| 70 | 60.2 | 63.9 | 67.0 | 71.0 | 78.8 |

| DIASTOLIC BLOOD PRESSURE MM HG | | SYSTOLIC BLOOD PRESSURE MM HG | | | |
|---|---|---|---|---|---|
| 80–84 | LESS THAN 120 | 120 TO 129 | 130 TO 139 | 140 TO 159 | GREATER THAN 160 |
| CALENDAR AGE | | REALAGE | | | |
| 35 | 30.6 | 33.6 | 35.0 | 36.3 | 40.6 |
| 55 | 49.4 | 52.7 | 54.7 | 56.8 | 62.8 |
| 70 | 62.8 | 67 | 69.1 | 72.2 | 79.3 |

| DIASTOLIC BLOOD PRESSURE MM HG | | SYSTOLIC BLOOD PRESSURE MM HG | | | |
|---|---|---|---|---|---|
| 85–89 | LESS THAN 120 | 120 TO 129 | 130 TO 139 | 140 TO 159 | GREATER THAN 160 |
| CALENDAR AGE | | REALAGE | | | |
| 35 | 33.0 | 35.0 | 36.0 | 37.1 | 41.0 |
| 55 | 51.6 | 55.0 | 56.4 | 57.8 | 63.2 |
| 70 | 65.5 | 70.0 | 71.6 | 73.3 | 79.9 |

(continued)

## Table 1.3

### The RealAge Effect of Combinations of Diastolic and Systolic Blood Pressure Readings (continued)

| DIASTOLIC BLOOD PRESSURE MM HG | | SYSTOLIC BLOOD PRESSURE MM HG | | | |
|---|---|---|---|---|---|
| 90–99 | LESS THAN 120 | 120 TO 129 | 130 TO 139 | 140 TO 159 | GREATER THAN 160 |
| CALENDAR AGE | | REALAGE | | | |
| 35 | 35.8 | 36.7 | 38.6 | 40.5 | 44.6 |
| 55 | 56.0 | 57.3 | 59.6 | 62.5 | 68.6 |
| 70 | 71.2 | 72.7 | 75.8 | 79.0 | 86.6 |

| DIASTOLIC BLOOD PRESSURE MM HG | | SYSTOLIC BLOOD PRESSURE MM HG | | | |
|---|---|---|---|---|---|
| 100 OR GREATER | LESS THAN 120 | 120 TO 129 | 130 TO 139 | 140 TO 159 | GREATER THAN 160 |
| CALENDAR AGE | | REALAGE | | | |
| 35 | 39.2 | 40.1 | 42.5 | 45.5 | 50.0 |
| 55 | 60.6 | 62.1 | 66.1 | 70.1 | 77.2 |
| 70 | 76.7 | 78.5 | 83.5 | 88.5 | 97.7 |

### For Women:

| DIASTOLIC BLOOD PRESSURE MM HG | | SYSTOLIC BLOOD PRESSURE MM HG | | | |
|---|---|---|---|---|---|
| LESS THAN 80 | LESS THAN 120 | 120 TO 129 | 130 TO 139 | 140 TO 159 | GREATER THAN 160 |
| CALENDAR AGE | | REALAGE | | | |
| 35 | 30.3 | 32.3 | 34.0 | 35.5 | 40.3 |
| 55 | 47.4 | 50.5 | 53.2 | 55.7 | 62.3 |
| 70 | 60.4 | 64.1 | 67.3 | 70.8 | 78.6 |

| DIASTOLIC BLOOD PRESSURE MM HG | | SYSTOLIC BLOOD PRESSURE MM HG | | | |
|---|---|---|---|---|---|
| 80–84 | LESS THAN 120 | 120 TO 129 | 130 TO 139 | 140 TO 159 | GREATER THAN 160 |
| CALENDAR AGE | | REALAGE | | | |
| 35 | 30.7 | 33.7 | 35.0 | 36.2 | 40.4 |
| 55 | 49.6 | 52.8 | 54.8 | 56.6 | 62.6 |
| 70 | 63.1 | 67.3 | 69.3 | 72.0 | 79.0 |

| DIASTOLIC BLOOD PRESSURE MM HG 85–89 | | SYSTOLIC BLOOD PRESSURE MM HG | | |
| --- | --- | --- | --- | --- |
| LESS THAN 120 | 120 TO 129 | 130 TO 139 | 140 TO 159 | GREATER THAN 160 |
| CALENDAR AGE | | REALAGE | | |
| 33.1 | 35.0 | 36.0 | 37.0 | 40.8 |
| 51.7 | 55 | 56.3 | 57.6 | 63.0 |
| 65.7 | 70 | 71.4 | 73.0 | 79.6 |

(CALENDAR AGE: 35, 55, 70)

| DIASTOLIC BLOOD PRESSURE MM HG 90–99 | | SYSTOLIC BLOOD PRESSURE MM HG | | |
| --- | --- | --- | --- | --- |
| LESS THAN 120 | 120 TO 129 | 130 TO 139 | 140 TO 159 | GREATER THAN 160 |
| CALENDAR AGE | | REALAGE | | |
| 35.6 | 36.8 | 38.4 | 40.2 | 44.1 |
| 56.0 | 57.0 | 58.9 | 62.1 | 68.0 |
| 70.9 | 72.3 | 75.4 | 78.5 | 86.0 |

(CALENDAR AGE: 35, 55, 70)

| DIASTOLIC BLOOD PRESSURE MM HG 100 OR GREATER | | SYSTOLIC BLOOD PRESSURE MM HG | | |
| --- | --- | --- | --- | --- |
| LESS THAN 120 | 120 TO 129 | 130 TO 139 | 140 TO 159 | GREATER THAN 160 |
| CALENDAR AGE | | REALAGE | | |
| 38.9 | 39.7 | 42.1 | 45.1 | 47.6 |
| 60.3 | 61.6 | 65.5 | 69.4 | 73.2 |
| 77.1 | 78.0 | 82.9 | 87.9 | 95.1 |

(CALENDAR AGE: 35, 55, 70)

mm Hg is the abbreviation for millimeters of mercury.

(assuming you were not overweight then—the "freshman 15" and the growing number of obese youths in high school and college are a recent phenomenon).

Next, measure your waist (the distance around at your belly button), and retake the measurements every few weeks, following these general guidelines:

1. Pull the measuring tape snugly around your belly button area, but do not allow the tape to compress the skin. If possible, use the same measuring tape for all current and future measurements.
2. When you measure yourself, take the measurements 3 times and record the median (the middle value, not average). Write your numbers down; it is

fun to watch them change as your RealAge workout program advances. Usually your waist size will get smaller before the numbers on the scale do. If you stick to your RealAge workout program, the changes you feel will be dramatic.

Why is your waist measurement important? Suppose, for example, that 3 months into your exercise program you find you have gained 2 pounds. On its own, this might be discouraging and you might want to give up. But your waist measurement might be several inches smaller. It could mean you have lost some body fat but have gained muscle. This is encouraging rather than discouraging, and of course it makes you younger.

Girth measurements can also help you estimate your body fat, and whether that fat is aging you. Fat cells around your hips don't cause aging, but fat cells in your abdomen secrete proteins that age your arteries and immune system. This arterial inflammation increases your risk for all the things aged arteries cause: heart disease, stroke, memory loss, impotence, and even wrinkling of your skin. Abdominal fat also contributes to diseases and conditions that decrease the quality of your life, such as diabetes, breast cancer, prostate cancer, arthritis, sleep apnea, and lower back pain.

Make sure to repeat the same tests in the same way in the future so that you can accurately assess the changes that have taken place in your body. I do these tests every 3 months and urge patients to pick an easy date to remember and do the same— January 15, April 15, July 15, and October 15.

## Exercise Capacity and Your Response

### *How Fast Can You Walk One Mile?*

All you need for this test is a watch with a second hand and a level surface on which to walk one mile. That could be eight to twenty city blocks, depending on how your city is built. If that's not convenient, go to your local high school (the tracks around football fields are usually one-quarter of a mile), or use a treadmill with a distance display. Whatever route you take, follow these instructions:

1. Warm up by walking at a moderate pace for 5 minutes.
2. Walk one mile as quickly as possible without causing pain or discomfort. (Do not run on this test, even if you can.)
3. Cool down by walking at a moderate pace for another 5 minutes.

Over the course of several months, if your time on the one-mile walk decreases, you have become more fit.

### Muscular Strength

The strength of a muscle is defined by the greatest amount of resistance it can over-come with one maximum effort. Because lifting with such a maximal effort can be risky, I recommend using a slightly lighter weight to gauge strength. Apply the test to three to five different upper body exercises and to two or three different lower body exercises (see Chapters 3 and 4 on strength training for exercises to choose from). Pick a weight that you estimate you can lift no less than 8 times and no more than 12 without losing form. Lift the weight as many times as you can without resting or stop-ping, then record the weight and the number of repetitions that you were able to do.

### Muscular Endurance

A muscle's endurance is defined by its capacity to exert a less-than-maximum force repeatedly over a period of time. Two standard tests are generally used: the push-up and the curl-up. You can compare your results for each test to established general-population norms or use them simply to gauge your individual progress.

## THE PUSH-UP TEST

The push-up test evaluates upper-body muscular endurance. Men should perform the test in the standard push-up position (*only* the toes and hands have contact with the floor). Women should assume a modified position, in which the knees also rest on the floor.

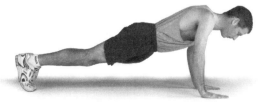
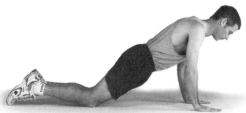

Whether you are male or female, remember to keep your spine straight and your head in line with your spine. Do not allow your back to sag or your buttocks to stick up in the air. Make sure to place your hands directly under or slightly wider than your shoulders. Lower your chest until it comes within 3 or 4 inches of the floor, and then push yourself back up. Inhale as you lower, and exhale as you push back up.

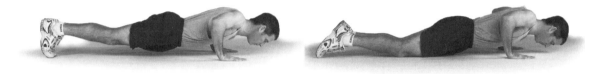

Follow these instructions:

1. Perform a 5-minute warm-up (walk at a moderate pace and do a few standing push-ups against the wall).
2. Assume the gender-appropriate push-up position.

### Table 1.4
### Usual Number of Push-ups at Various Calendar Ages*

| CALENDAR AGE | NUMBER OF PUSH-UPS FOR | |
| --- | --- | --- |
| | TYPICAL MAN | TYPICAL WOMAN (MODIFIED PUSH-UPS) |
| 20–29 | more than 35 | more than 18 |
| 30–39 | 25–29 | 13–19 |
| 40–49 | 20–24 | 11–14 |
| 50–59 | 15–19 | 7–10 |
| 60–69 | 10–14 | 5–10 |
| 70–79 | 6–9 | 4–10 |
| 80–89 | 3–5 | 2–6 |
| 90–99 | 1–3 | 1–4 |

* Norms are not ideals; more than typical is better.

3. Count the number of push-ups you can perform with proper technique. (You may rest during the test but only in the "up" position.)
4. Record the number of push-ups completed.

## THE CURL-UP TEST

The curl-up test evaluates abdominal muscular endurance. Both men and women perform the exercise in the same manner. Follow these instructions:

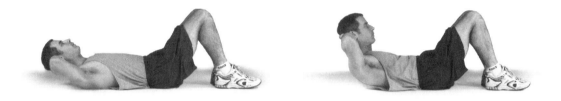

1. Warm up for 5 minutes by walking at a moderate pace and tightening your abdominal muscles a few times.
2. Lie on your back with your knees bent 90 degrees and your feet flat on the floor. Place your hands behind your head, and keep your elbows wide.

### Table 1.5
### Usual Number of Curl-ups at Various Calendar Ages

| CALENDAR AGE | NUMBER OF CURL-UPS IN 1 MINUTE FOR | |
| --- | --- | --- |
| | TYPICAL MAN | TYPICAL WOMAN |
| 20–29 | more than 45 | more than 35 |
| 30–39 | 30–34 | 25–29 |
| 40–49 | 25–29 | 20–24 |
| 50–59 | 20–24 | 15–19 |
| 60–69 | 15–19 | 10–14 |
| 70–79 | 10–14 | 7–9 |
| 80–89 | 6–9 | 4–6 |
| 90–99 | 2–5 | 1–3 |

3. Lift your head, shoulders, and shoulder blades off the floor. Then return to the starting position.

4. Perform as many curl-ups as possible in a minute.

5. Record the number of curl-ups completed.

### *Flexibility*

Your degree of flexibility corresponds to your capacity to move each of your joints through a full and normal range of motion. Adequate flexibility is essential for optimal functioning. Excessive flexibility can lead to unstable, injury-prone joints. I have selected a few important joints for you to evaluate. Before you take these tests, warm up with a brisk 5-minute walk or ride on a stationary bike.

### LOWER BACK

#### *Test #1: Trunk Flexion*

1. Sit on the floor with your feet about a foot apart and legs straight out in front.

2. Place one hand on top of the other with your fingertips lined up together.

3. Exhale and lean forward, extending your hands between your feet, with your fingertips almost touching the floor. (Keep your knees straight.)

Women 45 and under should be able to reach 2 to 4 inches past your feet. If you are 46 or older, you should be able to reach the soles of your feet.

Men age 45 and under should be able to reach the soles of your feet. If you are 46 or older, you should be able to come within 3 to 4 inches of the soles of your feet.

If you have less than the desired flexibility, make a note to be sure to include lower back stretches in your workout. (See pages 52–53 in Chapter 2.)

#### *Test #2: Trunk Extension*

1. Lie on your stomach with your hands in pre-push-up position.

2. Trying to maintain contact between your hip bones and the floor, slowly

press your chest off the floor. Do not force yourself into any discomfort. Stop pressing upward once the hip bones begin to leave the floor.

You should come close to straightening your arms with the hips still in contact with the floor. If you have less than the desired flexibility, make a note to be sure to include abdominal stretches in your workout. (See page 54 in Chapter 2.)

## HIPS

### *Hip Flexion Test*

1. Lie flat on your back with your arms at your sides and your legs straight out on the floor.
2. Without moving your hips or pelvis, lift your right leg up toward the ceiling, keeping your knee straight and keeping your left leg straight out on the floor.
3. Repeat with your left leg.

You should be able to lift your leg until it is pointing almost directly toward the ceiling (85–90 degrees of hip flexion). If you have less than the desired flexibility, make a note to include hamstring stretches in your workout. (See pages 37–39 in Chapter 2.)

### *Where Do You Want to Go?*

You've taken the tests and recorded the results on your progress sheet, so now you know exactly where you currently stand on your fitness map. But what do you do from here? In *Alice's Adventures in Wonderland,* when Alice asked a similar question of the Cheshire Cat, he came back with a crafty answer: "That depends a good deal on where you want to get to."

When you were a kid, you were active for the sheer joy of it. That's probably no longer the case now that you're an adult. Instead, chances are good that you're looking to increase your activity because you want a specific result. So decide why you want to exercise and write it down. You may have one reason, or you may have several. Your reasons will guide your journey. They will help you discover and reach your personal Point B.

*Translating Your Goals into "Body" Language*

People often state goals using language that does not specify concrete goals. Examples:

> *"I want an athletic build."*
> *"I want to feel better."*
> *"I want heads to turn this summer when I walk down the beach in my leopard-print bikini."*

These terms are colorful but imprecise because they do not give you concrete goals. It's hard to act on vague rhetoric. Let's translate some goals.

### I WANT TO LOSE WEIGHT.

Most often this statement really means, "I want to decrease the amount of fat in my body while maintaining or increasing the amount of muscle." This goal translated into an exercise strategy is: "Increase physical activity by walking 30 minutes every day, then add resistance training by lifting weights for 10 minutes, 3 times a week, and then add stamina-building activities." You wouldn't be wrong to write down "weight loss" as a goal. Weight loss, especially abdominal (or, more precisely, omental and organ) fat weight loss, will factor into each assessment of your progress. (When we refer to abdominal fat in the rest of the book, we mean omental and organ fat, or fat that causes you to age.) Just be sure that you know what you are actually referring to. We'll write down the "I want to lose weight" goal this way:

*Physiological meaning:* I want to decrease my abdominal and body fat and increase my muscle mass by making my waist thinner by an inch a month or by losing a pound a week for 4 weeks, and then by losing 2 pounds every month.

*Action Strategy:* Increase physical activity, resistance training, and stamina-building activities.

That action strategy can benefit almost everyone, and is the foundation of the RealAge Workout. But you may want more from your workout than just losing weight. You can tailor your plan to give extra time to certain activities after you've mastered the basic elements. For example, you might say:

## I WANT TO BE ABLE TO KEEP UP WITH MY GRANDCHILDREN.

*Physiological meaning:* I want to increase my energy level, make my arterial RealAge younger, and increase endurance.

*Action Strategy:* Put extra focus on stamina after resistance training.

## I WANT TO DECREASE MY RISK OF OSTEOPOROSIS.

*Physiological meaning:* I want to increase or maintain bone density, or make my bones younger.

*Action strategy:* Put extra focus on resistance training and weight-bearing physical activities.

---

### Question: Why do you call it "omental" fat as opposed to just abdominal fat?

Answer: Technically, abdominal fat can be just below the skin. That fat, called subcutaneous fat, doesn't age you much. Abdominal fat that can age surrounds your organs or stomach, also called omental fat. It is this omental and organ fat (so-called beer belly fat) that secretes proteins that make you older. That is right: Fat is in cells, and the fat cells surrounding the organs secrete stuff that is different in magnitude and effects than that secreted by fat cells at your hips or in your subcutaneous (just below the skin) tissue.

---

## I WANT TO IMPROVE MY GOLF GAME.

*Physiological meaning:* I want to improve my neuromuscular coordination, increase the strength in the muscles used for golf, and improve my flexibility.

*Action Strategy:* Put extra focus on spinal stabilization and functional exercises for 10 minutes every other day, balance training, resistance training with free weights, and daily stretching or yoga.

## I WANT TO TONE UP MY BODY.

*Physiological meaning:* I want to increase my muscular strength and size, and decrease my abdominal body fat.

*Action Strategy:* Put extra focus on resistance training.

## I WANT TO HAVE MORE CONTROL OVER MY DIABETES.

*Physiological meaning:* I want to decrease my body fat, increase my cells' sensitivity to insulin, and decrease arterial aging.

*Action Strategy:* Put extra focus on any physical activity, resistance activities, and stamina building.

Translating your reasons for exercising into words that describe specific physical processes will help you meet your goals.

Decide which factors should change, recognize your reasons for exercising, and set goals (a Point B) in relation to the chosen factors. Use the progress sheet on page 24 to set and chart your goals.

As you determine your goals, be realistic. For example, losing 10 pounds in 2 weeks is not realistic, not healthy, and not sustainable. Yes, you can do it with a crash diet, but I don't recommend this route. The overwhelming majority of people I questioned who did lose weight by such crash diets weighed around 10 pounds more within 3 months of ending their diet than they did before they started the diet. But you can lose a pound a week in a way that is healthy, and you can sustain a program of losing a pound every other week for many weeks.

Also, set short-term goals. Long-term goals such as "I will lose 50 pounds this year" do little to motivate you today. Keep your long-term goals in the back of your mind, but break them up into manageable steps that you can accomplish short term.

### Getting to the Point

The joke's an oldie, but a goodie: A visitor to New York stops a policeman and asks, "How do you get to Carnegie Hall?" The policeman answers, "Practice, practice, practice!"

So how are you going to get to Point B? The answer: plan and practice! This may require some experimentation. No one, not even the most knowledgeable fitness professional, knows how long it will take to achieve any given goal. Almost inevitably, you will over- or underestimate the amount of exercise and/or time it requires. That's fine. Not to worry. This is a creative process.

Based on our best knowledge of optimal exercise principles, make a plan that you think will work for you. Then—and this is key—set aside time to do it. Whether you decide to walk every day and do additional exercise every day or every third day— make it a priority. **Put it on your schedule and then do it.**

Ideally, you should consult with a personal trainer first and then periodically—say, every 3 months—see him or her again to observe your form. But too often the trainers want you to do all three forms of physical activity right from the start, and that's not in keeping with the philosophy of the RealAge Workout. Only work with a trainer who understands this fundamental principle, and who wants to be a true teacher, not just a taskmaster.

If it's not possible to get such a trainer, apply the principles we have discussed, look at your form in the mirror, and ask a friend to observe you. You will eventually get it right, and in the process you will become better and better at knowing how to get where you want to go.

## Point B: Is It the End?

When you set your Point B, keep in mind that your body and your life circumstances constantly change; Point B will be more of a way station than an ultimate destination. If all goes well, you'll reach many Point Bs on your journey, at which time you will assess your progress and determine where you want to go from there. (Be sure to pause when you get to a new Point B and celebrate.) But also know that when you hit a Point B, it immediately becomes your new Point A. New destinations, more successes, and even better celebrations await you.

We cannot describe or define the goal-setting process for every individual. It differs from person to person. But:

- ■ Never stop setting goals.
- ■ Make sure your goals reflect your desires and meet your standards of progress.

# Location and Destinations

| | POINT A | FIRST POINT B | SECOND POINT B | THIRD POINT B |
|---|---|---|---|---|
| Date | / / | / / | / / | / / |
| Where You Are: Your Weight | | | | |
| Heart Rate Resting | _____ | _____ | _____ | _____ |
| Blood Pressure | ___/___ | ___/___ | ___/___ | ___/___ |
| Waist Size | _____ | _____ | _____ | _____ |

## MUSCULAR AND FLEXIBILITY TESTS

| Date | / / | / / | / / | / / |
|---|---|---|---|---|

**Upper Body Strength**

| Body Part: | _____ | | | |
|---|---|---|---|---|
| Weight | _____ | _____ | _____ | _____ |
| Reps | _____ | _____ | _____ | _____ |
| Body Part: | _____ | | | |
| Weight | _____ | _____ | _____ | _____ |
| Reps | _____ | _____ | _____ | _____ |
| Body Part: | _____ | | | |
| Weight | _____ | _____ | _____ | _____ |
| Reps | _____ | _____ | _____ | _____ |
| Body Part: | _____ | | | |
| Weight | _____ | _____ | _____ | _____ |
| Reps | _____ | _____ | _____ | _____ |
| Body Part: | _____ | | | |
| Weight | _____ | _____ | _____ | _____ |
| Reps | _____ | _____ | _____ | _____ |

**Lower Body Strength**

| Body Part: | _____ | | | |
|---|---|---|---|---|
| Weight | _____ | _____ | _____ | _____ |
| Reps | _____ | _____ | _____ | _____ |

Body Part: _____
Weight _____ _____ _____ _____
Reps _____ _____ _____ _____

Body Part: _____
Weight _____ _____ _____ _____
Reps _____ _____ _____ _____
Push-ups _____ _____ _____ _____
Curl-ups in 1 min. _____ _____ _____ _____
Hip Flexion _____ _____ _____ _____
Trunk Extension _____ _____ _____ _____
Trunk Flexion _____ _____ _____ _____

**STAMINA TESTS**

How fast walked a mile _____ _____ _____ _____

**To Be Completed in Phase 4**

Maximum Heart Rate
  with Exercise _____ _____ _____ _____
Maximum Kcals per
  Minute _____ _____ _____ _____
Heart Rate Recovery
  2 Minutes after Exercise _____ _____ _____ _____

■ Keep your goals realistic and manageable, dividing them up into smaller pieces when necessary.

■ Set aside a specific amount of time in your schedule to focus on achieving your goals.

Now that you have your Point A, it's time to begin the journey. Along the way, you'll discover the magic of the RealAge Workout. And get ready to enjoy new vitality and energy, witness a change in the shape of your body, and not just feel—but actually be—younger. That's the RealAge promise. This program has transformed the lives of hundreds of RealAge patients, and it's going to do the same for you, too. I'd like to share the story of one of them to inspire you on your journey.

# Cynthia W.: A RealAge Workout success story

Cynthia W. was 43 when she became my patient after a heart attack scare. At 5 feet, 5 inches, she was 80 pounds heavier than she had been at age 18. Her waist was 41, well over the cutoff point for being overweight, and her RealAge was 55. As the managing editor of a business magazine, she had a chaotic job. When deadlines neared, she worked around the clock, living on take-out food and never leaving her desk. I immediately suspected the RealAge Workout could have a positive effect on Cynthia's health and well-being (but even I didn't know the amazing changes that were in store for her).

Cynthia told me, "One day, I woke up and I was 5 times the size I always thought I was. I don't want to haul all this weight around anymore. Tell me what I can do."

I told her I thought she should give the RealAge Workout a try, and explained how the regular physical activity of the program would not only help her lose weight and gain a smaller waist size but also help prevent arterial aging, and might protect her against future health challenges.

"I know I should go running, but I never do," she said, looking guilty.

"Don't worry. The RealAge Workout doesn't call for such strenuous activity right away," I told her. "Just start with Phase 1, which means that you'll be walking for 30 minutes every day—no exceptions, no excuses. Start with less if you need to, but slowly build up to 30 minutes."

Cynthia started her first "workout" that day. She walked from her house to the end of the block and back. That was it: short, sweet, and slow. The next day she did it again. By the end of the next week she was walking all the way around the block. Within 3 weeks, she was walking 8 city blocks—the equivalent of a mile—each day. Then she began timing herself, increasing her pace a little bit each time. Within 3 months she was walking half an hour each day and enjoying the results.

"I never thought I'd say this," she said to me one day, "but I actually find myself craving my daily walk. Me, the living paperweight, actually wanting to exercise!"

Cynthia had discovered that exercise doesn't have to be painful or exhausting. It can be something to look forward to, a treat. Energy-giving. She started doing it the easy way, remembering that health should be a priority—a fun priority—and soon she was ready to enter Phase 2: strength training of the foundation muscles. She started 10 minutes of weight lifting a day, working with a trainer for six sessions to get her form right. (It's wise to work with a trainer for a while, since improper weight lifting can cause injury.) Phase 3: strength training of the non-foundation muscles came next.

But then, when it was time for her to enter Phase 4, stamina exercise, Cynthia stalled. Although she was religious in her daily walks and weight lifting, she realized that because she did not enjoy the time she spent on the stationary bike that she owned, she wasn't doing a lot of vigorous exercise.

Then a breakthrough occurred. While on a business trip in November, she stayed in a hotel that had an exercise club with an elliptical trainer in front of a TV (she had not allowed herself to go to a health club until then because she had been less than proud of her body, she told me). She loved the elliptical trainer.

She treated herself to a big gift for Christmas: She bought an elliptical trainer for her home. With regular stamina exercise, Cynthia has been able to strengthen her heart, lungs, and arteries and increase her overall endurance. She continues to do 30 minutes of walking every day and 10 minutes of strengthening and flexibility exercises every day, which are especially important as she builds more stamina, since they help prevent injury.

Over the course of several years, as a result of following both the RealAge Workout and the eating plan outlined in *The RealAge® Diet,* Cynthia has transformed her body and her health. She has dropped 85 pounds, her waist is now 28, she lowered her blood pressure, and she feels a whole lot better. "I have more energy, and stressful events do not bother me as much; they just aren't as stressful anymore," she says with a laugh.

Cynthia has also found the love of her life. Her fiancé committed to letting her have at least an hour every evening to exercise; she needs only 30 minutes 3 times a week and 10 minutes on the other days, she told me, because she walks 30 minutes with two of her columnists at work, discussing business as they walk. In fact, she thinks the columns and ideas are crisper due to these walking meetings.

I have never seen anyone quite as happy to see me as Cynthia at her yearly planning and review session. She could be the poster child for RealAge: She has transformed herself from a 43-year-old with the energy and thoughts of a 55-year-old to someone who thinks, acts, and looks like she is 36 (her new RealAge).

The RealAge Workout really has done wonders for Cynthia and it can do wonders for you, too. So let's get started.

# Phase 1 (Days 1–30): Walking

## Can You Keep a Secret?

N o? That's great! Because I want you to share with everyone the biggest health secret I've learned from my patients—walking is the fountain of youth. It's the single best thing you can do for your health.

In the first RealAge book, I revealed that scientific studies had shown that walking alone gets you 40 percent of the total health benefit of all exercise. Yes—simple walking has that great an effect on your body. And during the year following the publication of that first book, I received about 150 thank-you notes and e-mails a day. (I still do.) For a doctor, it doesn't get much better than that, particularly since those notes and e-mails all contained a secret. People who succeeded in feeling more energetic sent me their secret; those that succeeded in losing weight sent me their secret; those that succeeded in quitting smoking also sent me their secret; and those that succeeded in lowering their blood pressure or getting their arthritis under control sent me their secret, too. And the secret for all was the same—30 minutes of walking every day. Most didn't walk fast, certainly not at the start. They walked at a comfortable pace, but they did it. And many were people who tried to reach impressive goals such as quitting smoking. They had failed in the past, but now they were reaching their goals simply by starting with a daily walk.

Walking is a wonder drug. It will make you healthier, more energetic, and younger. Sounds too good to be true, doesn't it? Well, you don't have to take my word for it. Have a look at the numbers:

### Table 2.1
### The RealAge Effect of Walking 30 Minutes a Day*

For Men:

| CALENDAR AGE | NO, OR LESS THAN 2 DAYS A WEEK | YES, 2 TO 6 DAYS EVERY WEEK | YES, EVERY DAY |
|---|---|---|---|
| | | REALAGE | |
| 35 | 35.8 | 35 | 34.3 |
| 55 | 57.3 | 55 | 53.9 |
| 70 | 71.7 | 70 | 68.1 |

For Women:

| CALENDAR AGE | NO, OR LESS THAN 2 DAYS A WEEK | YES, 2 TO 6 DAYS EVERY WEEK | YES, EVERY DAY |
|---|---|---|---|
| | | REALAGE | |
| 35 | 35.8 | 35 | 34.2 |
| 55 | 57.4 | 55 | 53.7 |
| 70 | 71.9 | 70 | 67.8 |

* These benefits or RealAge effects are for walking alone, and exclude the benefits of blood pressure reduction, heart rate reduction, stress reduction, better blood sugar and blood lipid control, its anti-inflammatory effects, etc. So the benefit is really much greater.

# Why Is Being Physically Active—That Is, Walking— So Good for the Body?

Two fundamental ways to maintain your health well until age 90 or 100 are keeping your cardiovascular and immune systems young. You can keep them young simply by engaging in regular physical activity. Let's look at how each one works.

### The Arteries

Simply put, you're as young as your arteries. When your arteries are not taken care of properly—when, for example, you do not do any physical activity—they get clogged with fatty buildup, diminishing their ability to dilate and constrict, and diminishing the amount of oxygen and nutrients that can reach your cells.

When your arteries clog with fatty buildup, not only does your cardiovascular system age quicker but your entire body does, too. Cardiovascular disease, which is brought on by aging of the arteries, is the major cause of heart attacks, strokes, many types of kidney disease, and memory loss. Even mild forms of non-lethal vascular disease can sap your energy and make you feel old and tired.

You may marvel at the 9-year-old boy who runs with boundless energy. He gets all that energy from his arteries, which expand in his active muscles, providing blood with more oxygen and other nutrients, and carrying away the waste products of metabolism. And the arteries that reach the inactive parts of his body constrict, allowing him to focus his energy where he needs it. So dilation and constriction of his arteries match the supply and demand of nutrients.

The hardening of your arteries leads to a loss of energy, wrinkling of the skin, impotence, and memory loss. The good news is that walking can help keep your arteries young and healthy.

### The Immune System

Physical activity also keeps your immune system younger. As you age, both your cell-based genetic controls and your immune system become more likely to malfunction. Those changes mean you are more likely to develop a cancerous tumor. Many types of arthritis are also examples of a breakdown of immune function. That's why arthritis is more common as you age.

Luckily, physical activity as simple as walking 30 minutes a day decreases the risk of such diverse conditions as arthritis, macular degeneration (a disease that lessens vision), and even cancer by an astonishing 50 percent compared to the non-exerciser. That's 50 percent.

Now that you understand how great walking is for your body and your health, you may be ready to dash out the front door. But wait! Before you go, there are a few more things about walking the RealAge way that you need to know.

### Do You Already Own What You Need?

- A watch. A watch is the single most important piece of fitness equipment you will own. Why? Because measuring your walking program by time is better than by distance. If you aim for a certain distance, you must find a track or a premeasured route, which is often inconvenient. Furthermore, if you attempt to run 3 miles or climb 1,000 stairs or do 10,000 steps, you are likely to force that amount upon your body. As a result, you are apt to overdo it if time pressured or walk slower if you have an open schedule. Just put 30 minutes of walking on your schedule, and then do it at a pace you enjoy. Can't do 30 minutes at a stretch? Get a watch with a cumulative stopwatch function and keep track throughout the day until you reach at least 30. (After a while you'll enjoy it so much you'll go past 30 on those days when you have enough time.)
- A good pair of walking shoes. Don't have any? Not to worry—go walking anyway. But before you finish 2 weeks of regular walking, carve out some time to get yourself a good pair of walking shoes.
- A calendar (even a Palm device with a calendar will do), both to schedule your daily walks and to check them off once you've accomplished them. Seeing the walk scheduled for a certain time in black and white will help you to remember that the walk must take priority every day. And checking off the days you stick to the plan will help you feel a sense of accomplish-

ment. Your accomplishments usually will motivate you to keep going. (At first when you mark "30-minute walk" on your calendar, it may feel like just one more item on your to-do list. But walking is addictive, in the best possible way. Before you know it, you'll be hooked. You'll find you can't wait to get out of the house or office for your daily walk.)

■ A pedometer (optional). Having a pedometer will help you go the extra distance when you're feeling great. You might consider buying yourself one as a reward for completing your first 30 days of walking. Because once you've accomplished that milestone and are in better shape, you may increase your pace (gradually) by doing more steps within that 30 minutes. It's fun to see how many more you do as your plan progresses.

### *You Will Have to Make Walking a Priority—Every Day, No Excuses*

You must make 30 minutes of walking a priority every day. And that's walking—not gardening, or house cleaning, or putting golf balls. You can do those things, too, but they can't take the place of your daily walk.

Some people—such as women busy with children—have told me they consider it selfish to spend time on themselves. But nothing is further from the truth. Exercising is a way of showing love for those you care about most. You will have more energy to care for them and you will be able to care for your children's children, rather than having your children spend time caring for you. We're becoming a nation of caregivers and care receivers; that's great, but if you want to be independent for a long time, start your walking program today.

### *You Will Need to Warm Up Before You Walk*

Warm-ups prepare your body, physically and psychologically, for the upcoming workout. When you warm up, you increase the blood flow in your muscles and increase your body temperature, two factors that make it possible for your body to achieve optimal performance.

Here's why: Muscles heated by a warm-up become less viscous and more pliable and flexible. This decreased viscosity makes them more mechanically efficient. It also lessens the chance of an injury. Warming up also helps the cartilaginous space in your joints enlarge with increased circulation of fluid. The increased space makes your joints more flexible and mobile.

A warm-up is any activity that satisfies the following conditions:

■ Increases your heart rate to at least 50 percent of its maximum (or at least 85 beats per minute, no matter what your age)

■ Increases your rate and depth of breathing

■ Elevates your body temperature

■ Utilizes the muscles you will use in the upcoming activity

■ Takes your joints through the full range of motion needed for the upcoming activity

---

### Can I warm up by simply turning up the thermostat, throwing on a wool body suit, tossing back a mug of hot cocoa, or sweating in a sauna for 10 minutes?

While these procedures might elevate your core temperature, none will cause your heart or breathing rates to increase sufficiently (unless, of course, you have company in the sauna). And they will not prepare the appropriate muscles or joints for what's coming.

---

For walking, a slower walk is the warm-up. Do so for several minutes—exactly how long depends on your age. As we become chronologically older, our bodies react more slowly to stimuli—see Box on page 35. You will know you are warmed up when you start to feel a little warmer and your heart beats a little faster.

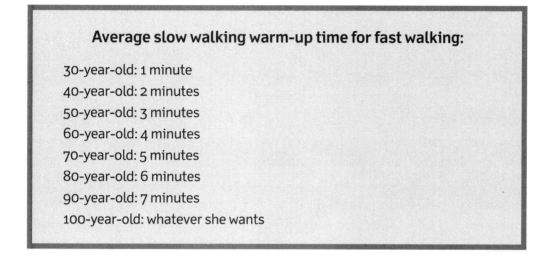

**Average slow walking warm-up time for fast walking:**

30-year-old: 1 minute
40-year-old: 2 minutes
50-year-old: 3 minutes
60-year-old: 4 minutes
70-year-old: 5 minutes
80-year-old: 6 minutes
90-year-old: 7 minutes
100-year-old: whatever she wants

### In the Beginning, You Will Need to Take It Easy

For most people, strenuous exercise is unpleasant. If you work so hard that you do not enjoy it, you will probably stop. We're talking complete stop. In addition, if you overdo it, you are likely to develop an overuse injury. You've heard the saying "No pain, no gain!" Fuggedaboutit. Pain is your body trying to tell you that you're doing something wrong. Do your body a favor and listen.

On the other hand, if you're feeling great, you can increase your activity, but **do not increase it more than 10 percent in any week, no matter how good you feel.**

### You Will Need to Stretch

Set aside 2 or 3 minutes to stretch when you're done. Stretching the muscles you just used allows them to be ready for the next time you want to use them. It is rumored to decrease soreness, but I cannot find hard evidence that supports that claim. But above all, stretching improves and maintains joint range of motion. Without a normal range of motion in the joints, daily activities become more difficult to perform and the risk of musculoskeletal injury increases. Great health without stretching is like trying to look good without combing your hair—it ain't gonna happen.

If you learn to enjoy it and indulge in it, stretching may become as much a benefit to your psyche as to your body. To perform a stretch, move slowly into the stretch position until you feel a gentle pulling sensation, not pain. Hold the stretch for 10 (a 30 count, the way most of us count) to 30 seconds (a 90 count) without bouncing. Multiple repetitions of stretches provide maximum benefit, so repeat each stretch at least twice or a third time if possible. If your schedule does not allow for multiple repetitions, perform each stretch once, but hold the stretch for at least 20 seconds. You need to do one stretch for each of the muscle groups you exercise.

Stretches should be felt in the muscle you exercised, not in a joint. If you feel pain in a joint when performing a stretch, stop immediately. Check your position and try the stretch again. If you still feel pain in the joint, discontinue that stretch immediately. You may end up stretching the joint capsule and/or other structures that keep the joint stable. Likewise, if you find yourself looking like a circus performer—having to contort and pull excessively in order to feel a stretch—you are either positioned incorrectly or you are flexible enough in that area and do not need to stretch further.

For a post-walking stretch, concentrate on the quadriceps, hamstrings, gluteals and piriformis (buttocks), adductors, hip flexors, calves, and lower back. It's not necessary to do them all, but you should choose at least one stretch per muscle group. If a given muscle group seems exceptionally tight, choose at least two of the stretches from that group or perform one of the stretches from that group several times. We've also put additional stretches for most groups on our Web site.

We've included photos (see pages 37–54) to help you see how you should look when you're doing the stretch correctly. A word about those photos. Tracy, my collaborator for this book, is also the model in many of them. Believe it or not, she's a mother of five, no, six, but who's counting? Let the photos of Tracy both instruct and inspire you as you begin to learn the stretches that will provide the perfect ending to your daily walk.

# HAMSTRING STRETCHES

The hamstrings are one group, but actually three different muscles that run up and down the back of your leg between your hip and your knee. These muscles (1) bend your knee, as if you were to kick your heel up behind you and (2) straighten (extend) your hip, as if you were bent forward with a straight back and wanted to lift yourself back upright. When you stretch this muscle group, you should feel the pull along the back of your thigh. If you feel it at the back of your knee instead, try bending your knee slightly or try one of the other hamstring stretches.

## STANDING HAMSTRING STRETCH

Place your foot up on an elevated surface with your knee straight but not locked. Lean forward from your hips, keeping your back as straight as possible, until you feel a gentle stretch in the back of your thigh. Keep your standing leg slightly bent. Repeat with the other leg.

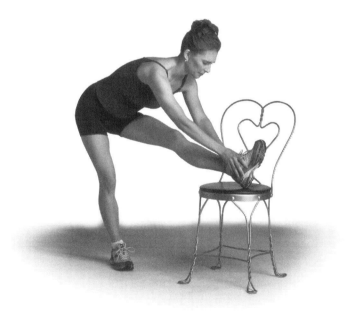

## SEATED HAMSTRING STRETCH

Sit on the floor with one leg bent and the other leg extended out in front of you. Lean forward over the straight leg, keeping your back as straight as possible, until a gentle stretch is felt along the back of your thigh. Repeat with the other leg.

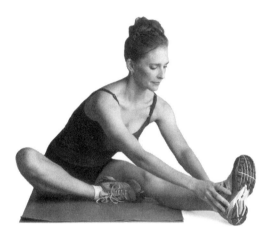

## LYING HAMSTRING STRETCH

Lie on your back with one leg extended straight out on the floor, the other leg extended up toward the ceiling. Place your arms at your sides or hold the back of your raised thigh. Pull the extended leg toward your head until you feel a gentle stretch along the back of your thigh. Do not allow your hips to tilt upward or your lower back to press against the floor. Try to keep the natural arch in your lower back. You will notice that this correct position prevents your leg from extending too far toward you. Repeat with the other leg. You may also perform this stretch in a doorway and rest your heel against the door frame.

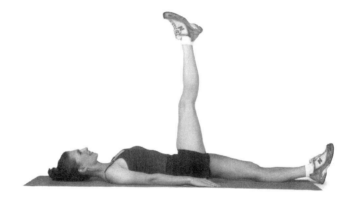

For all hamstring stretches:

- Never lock your knees.
- Make sure to maintain a straight back.
- Bend your leg if you feel pain or pulling in the back of your knee.
- Never bounce.

## QUADRICEPS STRETCHES

The quads, as they are often called, consist of four muscles that run along the front of your thigh. These muscles both (1) straighten your knee, as if you wanted to kick someone sitting across from you at the table, and (2) bend your hip, as if you were in a high-kick chorus line. When you stretch this muscle group, you should feel it along the front of your thigh. If you sense discomfort in your knee, try straightening your knee a little more and pressing forward more with your hip, flattening the crease at the front of your upper thigh.

### STANDING QUADRICEPS STRETCH

Stand on one leg. Bend the other leg and reach back to grab your ankle behind you. Point your knee down toward the floor so that your thigh is vertical and your shoulder, hip, and knee are in a straight line. Press your hips forward (tuck your pelvis under), extending the hip, until you feel a gentle stretch along the front of the thigh. Repeat with the other leg.

Variation: If you cannot grab your ankle or find it uncomfortable, stand with your back to the side of an armchair or stool and prop your foot on the armrest behind you instead of holding it with your hand.

Tips: Keep your foot directly behind you; do not pull it to one side. Do not pull your foot too close to your buttocks.

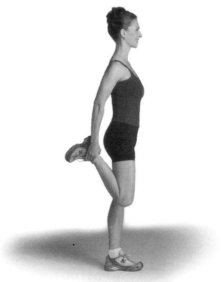

## LYING QUADRICEPS STRETCH

Lie on your side. Bend your top leg and reach back to grab your ankle behind you. Press your upper hip forward (tuck your pelvis under), extending the hip so that your shoulder, hip, and knee are in a straight line. Continue extending the top hip (pressing it forward and tucking your pelvis under) until you feel a gentle stretch in the front of your thigh. Repeat with the other leg.

Tip: Do not pull your foot upward or pull your foot too close to your buttocks; this places stress on the knee joint.

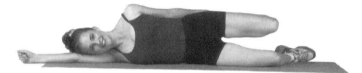

## PIRIFORMIS AND BUTTOCKS STRETCHES

The piriformis is a relatively small muscle that runs almost horizontally between your lower back (sacrum) and your hip. It rotates your hip to the outside, as if you were to lift your leg slightly and turn your leg so that your toes point outward. It helps stabilize your hip during many activities and can get quite tight, especially in runners. If your piriformis becomes tight or spasms, it can cause great pain by irritating the sciatic nerve that runs through it. When you stretch your piriformis, you should feel the stretch at the base of your buttocks.

### STANDING PIRIFORMIS STRETCH

Grasp a door frame, a pole, or something stable you can pull on. Cross one ankle above the opposite knee. Bend the standing leg and drop your hips down toward the floor and back behind you. Keep dropping your hips down and back until you feel a gentle stretch under the thigh and in the buttock of the lifted leg. Repeat with the other leg.

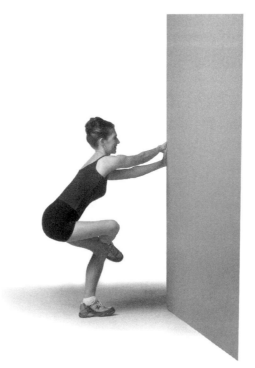

## SEATED PIRIFORMIS STRETCH

Sit on the edge of a chair or bench and cross one ankle over the opposite thigh. Lower your knee to the outside and toward the floor as you lean slightly forward from your hips. Keep the natural arch in your lower back. Continue leaning forward and dropping your knee until you feel a gentle stretch under the thigh, hip, or buttock of the crossed leg. Repeat with the other leg.

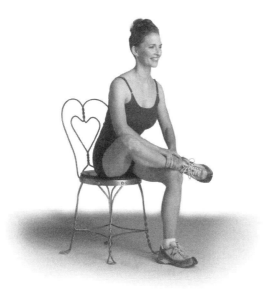

## LYING PIRIFORMIS STRETCH

Lie on your back and bend one leg, placing the foot flat on the floor. Cross the ankle of your other leg just above the opposite knee. Lift your foot off the floor and bring both legs toward your chest. You may hold on to your thigh to help pull your legs toward you. Continue drawing your legs toward your chest until you feel a gentle stretch near the hip and buttock of the leg that is closest to you. Repeat with the other leg.

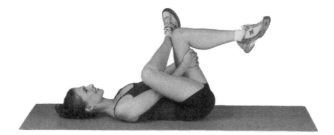

# ADDUCTOR/GROIN STRETCHES

This muscle group consists of six muscles located along the inner thigh, mainly toward the top of the thigh. These muscles rotate your hip inward and bring your leg toward the midline of your body. They are the muscles you would use to cross one leg over the other, but they function primarily as stabilizers in activities involving squatting or lunging such as skiing.

## STANDING LEG TO THE SIDE STRETCH

Stand and lift one leg out to the side, placing your elevated foot on a bench or chair with your toes and knee pointing upward. Keep the elevated leg straight, but do not lock your knee. Bend your standing leg slightly and lean your upper body forward a little, hinging at your hips. Keep the natural arch in your lower back. Continue to bend the standing leg until you feel a gentle stretch on the inside of your lifted thigh. Repeat with the other leg.

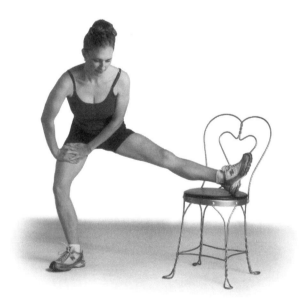

## LYING BUTTERFLY STRETCH

Lie on your back on the floor. Bend both knees and open them out to the sides, placing the soles of your feet together. Pull your feet in toward you until you reach a comfortable position. Keep the natural arch in your lower back, but do not arch excessively. Allow your knees to drop toward the floor until you feel a gentle stretch in the groin/inner thigh area.

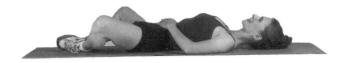

# HIP FLEXOR STRETCHES

The hip flexors are a group of six muscles along the front of the hip and thigh that flex or bend the hip. This bending can be caused in two main ways: the muscles can (1) cause a bent or straight leg raise as in a high chorus-line kick, or they can (2) help you perform a full sit-up by bringing your torso toward your legs when you are lying down. The hip flexors are often tight, especially in people who spend large amounts of time sitting. The stretch should be felt along the front of your hip.

## STANDING STRETCH

Stand in a comfortable position with one foot in front of the other. Center your weight between both feet. Keeping your back straight, bend your knees slightly to lower yourself toward the floor while tucking your hips (pelvis) under. Tuck your hips under until you feel a gentle stretch along the front of your hip (of the leg that is behind you). Repeat with the other leg.

Tip: Move your back foot farther back if you don't feel a stretch.

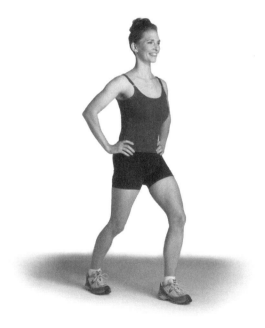

## KNEELING STRETCH

Kneel on the floor and place one foot flat on the floor in front of you. Keep your back straight and support yourself by resting your hands on the front thigh. Do not allow your front knee to extend forward past your toes. Extend your hip by moving your back knee a little farther behind you while tucking your pelvis (hips) under. Continue to reach back with your knee or tuck your hips under until you feel a gentle stretch along the front of your hip. Repeat with the other leg.

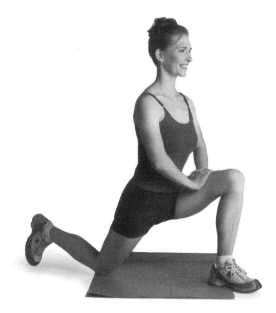

# CALF AND SOLEUS STRETCHES

This massive muscle group consists of two main muscles, the gastrocnemius and the soleus, which are located on the back of your lower leg. These muscles are often tight and should always be part of stretching after walking. Tight calf muscles can contribute to the common ailments of plantar fasciitis, which causes pain on the bottom of your foot, and Achilles tendonitis, which is associated with soreness in the back of your leg near your foot.

## STANDING LUNGE STRETCH

Stand with your hands against a wall. Reach one foot straight back to the floor behind you and bend your front leg to form a lunge position. Lean forward with your upper body and press your back heel down on the floor with the knee straight (not locked) until you feel a stretch in the back of your lower leg. Repeat with the other leg.

Variations: If you need a stronger stretch, reach the leg farther back behind you or move the front foot closer to the wall and lunge deeper. For a stronger soleus stretch, perform the above stretch but bend the back leg.

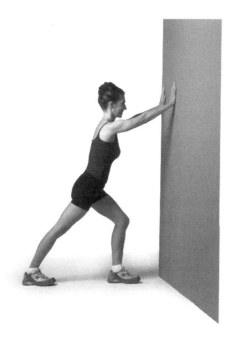 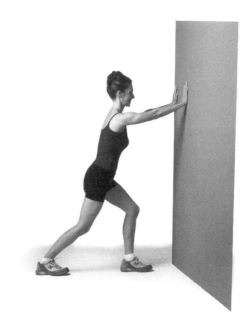

## STANDING TOES AGAINST WALL STRETCH

Stand close to a wall, tree, or the like and place the ball of one foot against it as high as possible while keeping the heel in contact with the floor. Keeping the leg straight, move your body and hips forward toward the wall until you feel a stretch in the back of your lower leg. To stretch the soleus, bend the knee of the leg that is against the wall. Repeat with the other leg.

Variation: You can also perform this stretch by hanging your heel off the edge of a curb or stair.

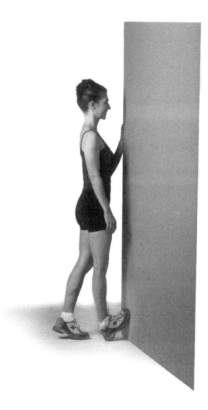

## SEATED ANKLE FLEX

Sit on the floor with both legs extended out in front of you, keeping your back as straight as possible. Pull your toes toward you until you feel a stretch in the back of your legs.

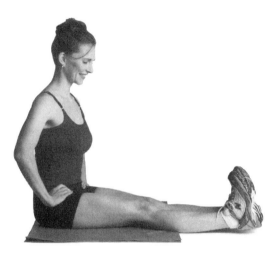

## LOWER BACK STRETCHES

Your lower back contains many muscles and joints. The complexity of these structures and their integrated nature as part of a whole system make lower back pain common and its cause hard to diagnose.

The following lower back stretches focus mainly on the extensors called the erector spinae. These lift your body back to an upright position if you are bent forward. Everyday activities such as leaning over to brush your teeth or filling a pot with water use these muscles. Even though you should feel this stretch mainly in your lower back, you may also feel it along your buttocks and the back of your upper thighs if you are tight in those muscles groups. I feel I need to reemphasize a key point here—as with other stretches, if you have pain in the area you want to stretch, check with a physician to make sure you can stretch safely; if the pain gets worse, discontinue the stretch and see your physician.

### STANDING FORWARD BEND

Stand with your feet hip width apart and knees slightly bent. Lower your head toward the floor first, followed by your shoulders and upper back. Curl your body forward and down one vertebra at a time. Allow yourself to hang down toward the floor. Bend your knees a little more and tuck your hips underneath as you slowly roll back up, one vertebra at a time, to a standing position.

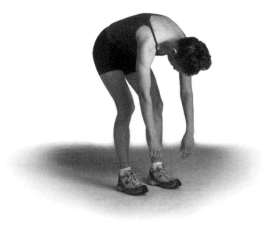

## CHAIR SEATED FORWARD BEND

Sit near the edge of a chair or bench with your legs a little more than shoulder width apart. Lean your upper body forward and allow yourself to hang down toward the floor.

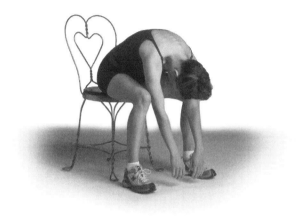

## FLOOR SEATED FORWARD BEND

Sit on the floor with your legs crossed. Lean forward with your upper body, reaching out in front of you with your arms. Keep your head in line with your spine.

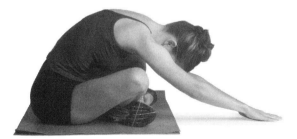

# ABDOMEN STRETCH (SPHINX AND COBRA)

The following stretches actually stretch the abdominal muscles (and the chest as well), but they benefit the back as much as they do the abdomen. These stretches are useful for maintaining the range of motion and the overall health of the back.

Lie on your stomach. Keeping your hips and legs on the floor, lift your head, chest, and rib cage off the floor. Support yourself by placing your forearms on the floor, palms facing down, with your elbows directly below your shoulders. Keep your head in line with your spine and your shoulder blades pulled together and down.

Variation: If you want a stronger stretch, press up onto your hands. You are not ready for this stretch, however, if your hips come up off the floor when you straighten your arms.

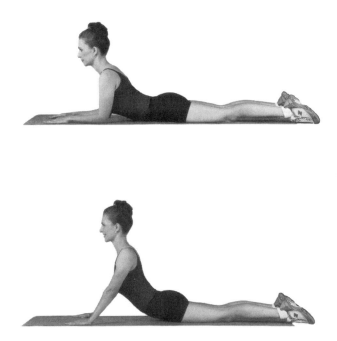

*Today Is the First Day of Your RealAge Workout Plan.*

Walking has provided our late-night comedians with some great jokes. One goes like this: *My neighbor started walking three miles a day when he was in his sixties. He just turned 96 and his kids have no idea where he is.* Funny—and the powerful effects of walking on your health will let you have even more fun for many tomorrows. Write to www.lettersto tomorrow.org about why you are starting your RealAge workout plan and share it with many.

I'm passionate about making you younger and letting you discover how good you can feel. But you need to take the first steps, and you must begin by walking—30 minutes a day, every day, no excuses. If you do that, I can virtually guarantee you'll feel better, have more energy, laugh more, and be younger for the rest of your life.

So let's get started. Mark your calendar, put on your watch and shoes, and then head out the front door to start your warm-up. You will be giving yourself (and your family) a great gift—a happier, healthier, more energetic you.

## FAQs About Walking

### Is it really true that I'm likely to live longer if I walk just once a week?

According to a July 2004 study in the *American Journal of Preventive Medicine,* older adults who exercised only once a week were 40 percent less likely to die in the next 12 years than those who did nothing at all. The study followed more than 3,200 men and women over the age of 65. After accounting for differences in age, education, smoking habits, and illnesses such as diabetes or hypertension, people who said they "exercise only occasionally" still had a 28 percent lower risk of dying during the 12-year study period than those who described themselves as inactive. That said, I don't want you to walk just once a week. I want you to walk every day. You'll feel and look better for it.

### Should I really aim for duration rather than distance in my daily walks?

Tight schedules rule our lives. For most of us, if it ain't on the schedule, it ain't gonna get done. Which means if you do not put physical activity on your schedule, your schedule will force physical activity out of your life and your RealAge will get older rather than younger. Only you know how much time you can devote to your workout. Whatever it is, schedule it in.

You may have 60 consecutive minutes each day or 10 minutes twice a day. Everyone can do at least 10 minutes a day. No one has ever admitted to me that he or she is so disorganized as to not be able to commit 10 minutes a day to exercise.

**If my spouse or family doesn't want to walk with me, won't I feel guilty taking the time for myself?**

*Doing physical activity such as walking is showing love for those you care about the most.* The exercises in *The RealAge® Workout* will strengthen your heart, arteries, and lungs; they delay—and may even reverse—arterial and immune system aging, and stress-induced aging. That means you'll have even more time with your loved ones in the long run.

Talk to your spouse and/or children about the need for physical activity and its importance for all of you. Each of you can set physical activity goals. When one of you reaches a goal, you can all celebrate together. *It may sound corny, but encouraging someone to stay in shape is the best way to say "I love you."* It means you want those people to be around for a long time. (See my restrictions for children and exercise on page 190 in Chapter 6.)

**What should I do in bad weather when I can't walk outside?**

There's nothing better than a brisk walk down a country road, a suburban street, or a city sidewalk, but if the weather doesn't cooperate, here are some alternatives.

- There are great clothes made for challenging weather conditions, and getting outside in bad weather can be surprisingly fun and refreshing.
- Malls are a terrific place to walk, and some of the more progressive ones have designated early morning hours just for walkers.
- Most Ys have walking tracks or treadmills that are comfortable and convenient, and the cost of joining a Y is usually reasonable.
- If you can afford one, buy a treadmill so that you can walk any time of day or night without even leaving the house.

Please let us know if you find other good spots. We would love to hear about them. (Write drmike@realage.com.)

**I get bored easily, especially when I walk. Any suggestions?**

Absolutely. Pick up a Walkman, an iPod, or a cell phone with a hands-free attachment. Make this the time to talk to friends or listen to your favorite radio program or the CD you never have time for. Pick up the audio version of a book you've been meaning to read, and "read" it in 30-minute increments. The new iPods, which contain more than 10,000 songs, are joys to behold. Slap on the earphones and the time might go so fast you'll be disappointed your 30 minutes are up. (Don't turn the music up too loud; you can hurt your ears. Time it and take an iPod break for at least 2 minutes of every 15.) Also try changing the scenery by varying your route. Look around you and try to notice new things each time you walk.

**I can't fit a 30-minute walk into my schedule; I'm in meetings all day.**

If you have trouble fitting a 30-minute walk into your schedule, try a business walk. Example: For one of your one-on-one meetings, take a paper and pencil along and turn it into a walking meeting. (If you are in better shape than your meeting partner, increasing the pace at which you walk will give you a serious negotiating advantage.)

**When I am ready to increase the speed of my walks, are there any rules I should follow?**

Yes—make sure you are walking for at least 30 minutes before you try to increase your pace. And then do so gradually. (If you increase your intensity too early, you may meet with discouragement and injury.)

**What is the minimum time a day spent walking?**

Thirty minutes—it can be in as small as 10-minute intervals, but no shorter. And 30 minutes is the secret.

**Thirty minutes a day of walking, and 10 minutes every other day of strength training, and 21 minutes three times a week of stamina seems like a lot. How can you call this "minimum work"?**

I am talking about the minimum to do for maximum benefit. So while it may seem like a lot of time, it's what you need for maximum benefit. Fit the walking into daily activities and you'll spend remarkably little extra time for extraordinary gains.

### I have a history of plantar fasciitis (a painful overuse injury affecting the sole of the foot). Can I walk?

Usually. If you are pain free now and have great walking shoes, go for it. But remember to ice your foot for 20 minutes every morning and night. You can do this using a bag of frozen peas covered with a plastic bag or a pliable, reusable cold pack that molds to your foot (available in the first aid section of most drugstores). After 20 minutes, stretch your foot and put the pack back in the freezer for future use. If you have had trouble or pain walking in the past, see a podiatrist and get fitted with the best walking shoes you can afford. Also consider taking two baby aspirins or half a regular aspirin with a glass of warm water before or after your walk. And remember to stretch your calves immediately following your walks.

### I already do stamina exercise such as jogging or swimming. Do I still have to start my RealAge workout with walking?

Yes. Even if you're already in great shape, adding that 30-minute walk every day will benefit you. However, readers who are already very active can tailor the plan as follows, if they choose (adding walking is not going backward—it really has proven to be a multiplying move to most of my patients):

1. Add 30 minutes of walking a day while continuing to do the level of stamina exercise that you are already used to.

2. Immediately add the foundation strengthening exercises if you are not already doing them.

3. Thirty days later, add the non-foundation muscle exercises unless you are already doing them, in which case keep doing them. (If you already are at maintenance—meaning you've already been strength training for 4 months or more—you can reduce the strength-training workout to once a week if you want to, but it will be a much tougher day.)

4. Then, in 30 days, increase the intensity of your stamina training to threshold, meaning that at least 1 minute out of every 7 of your routine, increase

(if you are not already doing so) to the absolute maximum intensity that you can. (I strongly recommend doing this only after 60 days of preparation so that you can have the strength in your muscles to protect yourself from injury.)

If you modify the plan in this way and find it's too tough, don't get discouraged. Just go back to square one and follow the plan exactly as it's outlined in the book.

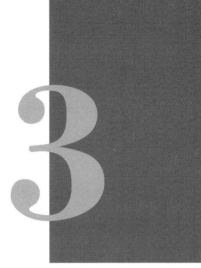

# Phase 2 (Days 31–60): Strengthening Your Foundation

Now that you've built up your energy supply chain and your contractile proteins by walking 30 minutes a day, every day, you're ready to start Phase 2. Those proteins are necessary so you do not injure yourself in this phase, where you will start strength training. This is an exciting new step in your RealAge journey. By strength training, you will make your RealAge younger by decreasing arterial aging, immune aging, and risk of disabling accidents. You will also make your bones stronger. Bone density normally decreases 5 percent every 10 years after age 35, making you more susceptible to the consequences of osteoporosis, lower back pain, hip pain, decreased functioning, and broken bones. But by strength training, you will keep your bones healthy and strong, and will reduce the risk of these debilitating conditions. In fact, you'll reduce such risks by over 80 percent.

Another wonderful result of strength training is that the muscle you will build is the best fat burner you can have. Body fat tends to increase with age. What's worse, a higher proportion of that fat finds its way by some awful magic to your abdominal area and around vital organs as if it were strangling them. Which is exactly what omental and organ fat (the fat that surrounds your stomach and intestines and other organs—we just call it abdominal fat) do. Like a creature from a horror story, abdominal fat transforms itself from a storage depot into a hormonal machine that secretes bad stuff that ages arteries, causing high blood pressure, high triglyceride levels, heart disease and type II diabetes, skin wrinkling, strokes, memory loss, decline in orgasm pleasure, and impotence. Without resistance exercises, your body replaces 5 percent of your muscle every 10 years with fat. But strength training just 30 minutes a week prevents this. Totally.

During this particular phase of your RealAge Workout, you will make your foundation strong and steady so that you can progress to Phase 3 with the least risk of injury. What, exactly, is your foundation? It is a set of muscles that, when you effectively train them, will make you strong at your body's core. Those sets of muscles are:

### 1. Central Abdominal Muscles

The central abdominal muscles consist of the transverse abdominis, running horizontally across your lower abdomen (in fact, it acts like a girdle to keep your abdomen flat); and the rectus abdominis, running vertically down the center of your abdomen.

### 2. Lateral Abdominal and Rotator Muscles

The lateral abdominal muscles are the internal and external obliques, which sit diagonally along the front and sides of your torso. The rotator muscles consist of both abdominal muscles and muscles along the spine that rotate or twist your torso.

### 3. Lower Back Muscles

Your lower back contains many muscles and many joints. The lower back exercises in this book focus mainly on the lower back extensors called the erector spinae. They lift your body back into an upright position if you are bent forward.

### 4. Buttocks, Quadriceps and Hamstring Muscles

The gluteus maximus is the major muscle of the butt. It forms the bulk of your backside, extends to the back of your upper thigh, and helps propel you forward when you are walking or running. The quads and hamstrings, at the front and back of the thigh, while not considered core muscles, are prime movers, and their strength is essential to having a great foundation and reducing the chance you'll develop hip or knee arthritis severe enough to immobilize you.

### 5. Upper Back Muscles

Your upper and middle back have a number of powerful muscles. They include the trapezius, the rhomboids, and the latissimus dorsi. These muscles run between your shoulder or shoulder blade and your spine. They allow you to shrug your shoulders, stand up tall by pulling your shoulder blades together, and pull something down or toward you.

### 6. External Rotators

The muscles at the top of your shoulder—including the infraspinatus and teres minor—are the rotators of the shoulder. They are the relatively weak muscles that allow you to rotate your hand and arm outward from your body.

### 7. Internal Rotators

These muscles, also relatively weak, and comprising the subscapularis group, allow you to rotate your shoulder and arm inward.

## The Warm-up for Strength Exercises

As with all types of exercise, you must warm up before engaging in strength training. I hate the word *must*, but you really must here. If you are doing only strength-building activities during today's RealAge workout and no stamina-building activities, begin with a general, whole-body warm-up (such as brisk walking), followed by lifting a much lighter weight through the same motion you'll be doing with the heavier one.

How long you should warm up depends on your age, as discussed in Chapter 2 (see Box, page 35).

## *What Equipment to Use?*

Resistance equipment includes any of hundreds designed to provide an opposing force to your muscles. As they work against resistance, your muscles get stronger. Most resistance equipment falls into three categories: weight machines, free weights, and rubberized (elastic) resistance devices. Each type possesses unique advantages and disadvantages.

## WEIGHT MACHINES

Weight machines vary greatly in price, quality, and design. If you have never practiced resistance training before, they can be a good way to start. You can learn proper form while increasing your strength. But soon after you begin your resistance program—certainly within a month or two—you should add free weights to the program.

### *Advantages of Weight Machines*

- They require relatively little skill and coordination. Because most machines "dictate" body position and movement, you achieve proper form with less practice than with free weights or rubberized resistance tubes.
- Well-designed machines may decrease the risk of injury.
- Many machines adjust to stronger and weaker points within a joint's range of motion, thereby strengthening the targeted muscle at all points in the range.
- Machines support and stabilize non-targeted body parts, while effectively isolating and strengthening targeted muscles. Most also facilitate optimal joint angles, thus promoting the most efficient workout for each particular muscle.
- Machines provide excellent resistance for lower-body work.
- You can easily track your weight-training progress.

*Disadvantages of Weight Machines*

■ Machines can keep the less than perfectly coordinated individual eternally clumsy, since they do not help you develop as much coordination as free weights.

■ Because machines isolate the working muscles and require no stabilizers to play their natural parts, they do not train the body well for the integrated movements that daily activities require. Cables and pulleys can be exceptions to this.

■ Certain machines, especially ones with few adjustable parts, may require you to assume a position not optimal for your joints and increase your risk of injury.

■ The more sophisticated and complicated machines can be intimidating.

■ Some machines are cumbersome and time-consuming to adjust from one exercise to another. (Manufacturers are decreasing this inconvenience factor.)

■ Machines usually are not made for small apartments and can be very expensive.

## FREE WEIGHTS

If you're looking for resistance equipment with no strings attached, free weights are for you. Dumbbells, barbells, and medicine balls—none are attached to a cable, pin, or pulley.

A dumbbell consists of a short handle placed between two bigger masses of weight. Dumbbells are used in pairs, and in spite of their name, are some of the smartest resistance equipment on the block. Barbells resemble dumbbells, but they are about 6 feet long. Most barbells are equipped with round, detachable, doughnut-shaped plates of varying weights. As a general rule, I prefer dumbbells, as the barbell can be problematic in some exercises such as the overhead triceps extension.

The medicine ball has been used for many years in sports and power training. It is making a strong comeback as functional weight training has gained popularity. (Functional strength training is moving a weight through a normal everyday motion, such as lifting a medicine ball as you'd lift and swing a bag of groceries.) Medicine balls are comparable in size to basketballs, although some measure a little larger or smaller, depending on material, construction, and weight. They weigh anywhere from 1 to 40 pounds. The ball's rubbery, often textured surface makes it easy to grasp. Some medicine balls are designed to bounce, enabling individuals to perform drills alone against a floor or wall. Some plop like a bag of sand when they hit the floor.

Regardless of type, all free weights work on the principle of constant resistance. That means the weight remains the same no matter what you do with it; the force providing resistance is nothing but good old-fashioned gravity. Therefore, the force that controls the weight is always moving toward the center of the Earth, or in more practical terms, toward the floor. **To take advantage of gravity's resistance, you must assume a position during each exercise that forces the targeted muscle to overcome gravity. To put it more simply, weights must move up because gravity is pulling them down.**

Let's look at a couple of examples. Bob and his friend Betsy both want to strengthen their chest muscles. Bob stands with a weight in each hand and holds the weights up and out to the sides, with his elbows bent 90 degrees, and then brings his arms together in front of him so that his forearms almost touch. He performs several repetitions, moving his arms out and together.

Betsy lies down on a weight bench and positions herself for chest flies (see page 112). She holds a weight in each hand with her arms extended toward the ceiling. She lowers her arms outward and down toward the floor, and then brings them back up toward each other again.

While both people are performing very similar movements, only Betsy is using gravity to her advantage by lying down. Bob uses his chest muscles to bring his arms forward, but gravity is not adding any resistance to this motion—not enough, at least, to matter. Bob's chosen exercise primarily strengthens his shoulder muscles, the muscles that must work to keep his arms lifted up. Even so, these muscles are only strengthened in a small part of their range of motion.

Therefore, before doing a free weight exercise, you must do the following:

1. Decide which muscle you want to work out.
2. Ascertain what movement that muscle makes.

## Question: Can I strength train if I have high blood pressure?

Answer: Strength training over the long run makes your arteries younger and more pliable, reducing blood pressure. But while you are actually doing the exercise, it raises your blood pressure and has even been associated with some rupture of aneurysms. The key is breathing in the right way. Breathing makes a difference, and here you should practice, practice, practice till perfect before lifting. Learn to exhale when you do the hardest part (the lifting for free weights) and you'll minimize (although not eliminate) the blood pressure rise. And this is one area where if you have a family history of aneurysm, you should check with your doc before you lift weights.

3. Position your body so that the weights move away from the floor when you perform the movement for that muscle.

Free weight trainers experience some of their best workouts lying down. If this idea appeals to you, consider buying a weight bench. If possible, purchase an adjustable bench that accommodates many positions. The seat back should allow you to lie flat, sit straight up, or at many angles in between, with your back fully supported. Even better, although not as essential, is a seat back that declines slightly, allowing your upper body to lie lower than your hips. Try a few. You may prefer a firm bench to a cushioned one, a narrow to a wide one, or a short to a long one. A stability ball may also be used like a bench for many of the free weight exercises.

*Advantages of Free-Weight Training*

■ Free-weight exercises simulate real-life activities more closely than other resistance exercises. The gallon of milk you just pulled out of the refrigerator is an 8-pound free weight. Your briefcase is a free weight. So is your pet, your child, even your telephone. When you strength-train using free weights, you strengthen the body in a functional way (especially in standing exercises); you become stronger and more efficient for the activities you perform each day.

■ Free weights are inexpensive and space efficient. You can buy as a block, or as a set of hexagonal dumbbells, consisting of pairs of 3-, 5-, 8-, 10-, 12-, 15-, and 20-pound weights, for under $80 (cast-iron alloy free weights cost about 50¢ a pound). Free weights can be kept under a bed, in a closet, behind a toy box or couch, in a bread box (perhaps the best use for a bread box), or on a space-efficient weight rack.

■ Free weight training improves your proprioception, balance, and coordination. Proprioception? Big word. Important function! Your body contains proprioceptors—nerve endings that help you judge where one body part is in space and in relation to other body parts. Proprioception allows you to walk down the stairs, catch yourself from falling, or bring a spoon to your mouth rather than to your nose.

■ With free weights, you can vary your joint position or range of motion, providing opportunity for sport-specific training or training with an injury or physical limitation.

■ Many free weight exercises require you to use multiple muscles for stability. Your foundation muscles support your torso and stabilize your spine during free weight activity. (Such stabilizers are not used as much with exercises done lying on your back or sitting fully supported against a bench.) But when these back stabilizing muscles are strong, they do just that—they protect your back.

■ Free weights provide almost unlimited variety. You (if you are typical) can do a dumbbell triceps exercise on your back, standing, sitting upright, or leaning forward in a bent-over position.

■ With free weights you can easily and quickly move from one exercise to another (no changing of pins, settings, attachment sites, or machines).

■ You can easily track your progress using free weights.

■ Dumbbells, one particular kind of free weight, force each side of your body to lift equal amounts of weight. Because each side works independently, dumbbell training helps detect and correct imbalances. For example, while performing a biceps curl, you may find that one arm begins to fatigue before the other. This signals an imbalance of strength that may be corrected by doing more work with your weaker arm or carrying your briefcase or garbage on your weaker side more frequently.

### Disadvantages of Free-Weight Training

■ A free weight accumulates momentum as it moves. As a result, injuries can occur when the force required to stop a free weight's momentum exceeds the forces that your muscles, bones, or joint structures can safely provide. Such injuries often occur when people are simply trying to get into or out of the starting or ending positions of an exercise. (Positioning is often more hazardous than actually doing the exercises!)

■ Safe and effective free-weight training requires a higher level of knowledge, skill, and concentration than weight-machine training. Some instruction in proper form and technique is critical, and you probably should lift free weights only when you will not be distracted, especially by kids or pets.

■ If you use extremely heavy weights, getting into your starting position may be difficult or dangerous. You can solve this problem by simply recruiting an exercise partner to help you (and enjoy the RealAge benefits that social interaction provides). But this is a disadvantage of free weights unless you have a willing (and able!) partner.

■ Free weights are less effective for lower-body work. If we were built like monkeys, we could pick up free weights with our feet (and do pull-ups with our tails), but most of us aren't.

## RUBBERIZED RESISTANCE

Rubberized resistance, stretch bands, or elastic resistance is made of surgical tubing and comes in a variety of shapes, colors, and strengths. The strength, or resistance, of a band depends on its thickness and its degree of displacement (how much the tubing is stretched). The thicker the tube and the more stretched, the greater the resistance. Unlike free weights that provide constant resistance through their range of motion, tubing provides varied resistance, often referred to as progressive resistance.

Because the resistance is supplied by the elastic or tensile properties of the equipment itself, gravity will not play a large role in your rubberized resistance workout. Even astronauts in space make effective use of rubberized resistance. With gravity out of the picture, you do not need to worry about positioning your exercises with respect to the floor or the center of the Earth. You simply anchor the tube to resist the action you intend. You need know only one thing to strengthen a specific muscle—which actions that muscle performs.

### *Advantages of Rubberized Resistance*

■ Tubing is portable, convenient, cheap, space efficient, and perfect for travel. A complete multilevel resistance set of tubing (different colors for different resistance), with all the trimmings, costs no more than $50.

■ Much like free weights, tubing leaves room for almost limitless variety.

■ Bands cater to individual physical idiosyncrasies and limitations by allowing variations in joint position and range of motion.

■ Tubing exercise causes a low rate of joint and muscle injury.

### *Disadvantages of Rubberized Resistance*

■ It is harder to track your progress in a precise way.

■ The resistance of each band may change slightly with use.

■ Since the more the tubing stretches the more its resistance increases, rubberized resistance strengthens each targeted muscle more at the end of its range of motion than at the beginning. As a result, a muscle may encounter its greatest resistance at a mechanically weak point in its range, when it would be preferable to meet with decreased resistance. Therefore you will not strengthen the muscle optimally and may be at increased risk of injury.

### USING YOUR OWN BODY WEIGHT AS RESISTANCE

I once worked with a client who refused to do any exercise that required equipment. We designed a workout plan that employed nothing but his body weight for resistance. Although not ideal, it helped him achieve a younger RealAge.

As with free weights, body weight exercises need gravity for resistance. You must keep this in mind as you position yourself.

Proper positions for these movements, especially for upper-body muscles, look like inverted renditions of comparative free weight exercises. For example, look at a dumbbell chest press (page 111). It requires lying on your back and pressing weights up and away from the floor. If you want to do the same movement without equipment, using only your body to strengthen the same muscles, you must lie on your stomach and push your body away from the floor (the common push-up). In each instance, the action of the arms is virtually the same.

To know if you are using your body weight appropriately, ask the following questions:

1. What muscle do I want to work?
2. What action does that muscle perform?
3. Does performing that muscle's action in this exercise position lift my body weight away from the floor?

If you answer yes to question 3, you are likely working the muscle you want.

### Advantages of Body Weight Exercise

■ Your body is free, accessible, and portable.
■ You can explore a variety of exercise positions to obtain different levels of resistance for the same basic muscles or to work different muscles. For example, some variations on a push-up theme include wall, tabletop, knee, basic, triceps, incline or decline, plyometric (rapid), and one-arm push-ups.
■ You can document your progress by noting the number of repetitions you can perform or your advancement to a more demanding position.

### Disadvantages of Body Weight Exercise

■ Back, shoulders, and biceps muscle groups need a bar or prop to be targeted.
■ Your body weight determines the amount of resistance available, and this might be either too much or not enough.
■ While it is difficult to compose an entire regimen of strength training just

with your own body, body exercises (especially sit-ups and push-ups) make up a necessary portion of almost all strength training programs.

### Which Types of Exercise Equipment Should You Use?

The answer lies both in where you want to work out and how much you can spend. Optimally, your workout should incorporate more than one resistance training modality, including machines, free weights, body weight exercises, and rubberized resistance.

If you want to work out at home, and you don't have much space or much extra cash, your "gym" may consist only of some tubing and a few dumbbell weights. If you have a little more space and can afford a bench, get it. (A set of free weights, some tubing, and a good bench are the staples of a resistance training program.)

If you have more space and money, you can invest in a larger home gym. Nirvana: The ability to work out at home and the liberty to choose between free weights, tubing, or machines, what could be better?

And if you work out at a health club, you'll probably have more equipment available than even Arnold Schwarzenegger could use in one day. But remember—as much as you love using those fancy machines at your health club, free weights and simple cable or pulley machines benefit you in some ways that other machines don't. You should use free weights or cables at least once a week.

### How Much Resistance Should You Use?

Whatever method you choose, you must determine the level of resistance (such as the weight of a free weight or the setting on a machine) that's appropriate for you for each exercise. Use the following rule: **If you can lift a weight or carry through a movement on a machine more than 12 times in the desired motion without feeling almost completely fatigued, you need a heavier weight or greater resistance. If you cannot lift it 8 times, you need a lighter weight or less resistance.**

This is the optimal way to train. However, if you are (1) frail, (2) still in your first 2 months of resistance training, (3) tend toward overuse injuries such as bursitis or tendonitis, or (4) have a RealAge older than 65, you must tailor the plan. You will likely benefit more from one set of 10 to 12 repetitions of each exercise with lighter weights, 3 times each week. After 2 months, you can increase your training by adding another set or adding a new exercise to your routine or by doing the same set at a slightly slower pace.

The reason you will want to start with light weights is that if you are frail, the connective tissues surrounding your joints need time to adapt to exercise. Even though your muscles may be able to handle a rapid weight progression, your tendons, ligaments, and other connective tissues may not. By keeping your weights lighter (5 to 10 pounds lighter) during the first 2 months of training, you may prevent the development of tendonitis, bursitis, and other overuse-related and stress-induced injuries. After 2 months, if you are feeling stronger, slowly start making the weights heavier.

## Your RealAge Foundation Exercises

For optimal strength training of your foundation, follow these rules:

1. You must choose at least one exercise from each of the seven foundation muscle groups in order to work that group. (Do not work out some of the muscle groups while neglecting others. Doing so can cause instability and invite injury.)
2. You must train each muscle group 3 times per week (twice a week at a minimum).
3. You must rest each muscle at least 48 hours to ensure recovery and repair. (If you want to do strength training every day, work out different groups on different days, letting the others recuperate. If you want to do strength training only 3 times a week, work out all groups on your strength-training day.)
4. Use equal weights for both sides of the body. Do not, for example, use a lighter weight for your left arm if that arm is weaker. (Instead, slowly build that muscle up to catch up to the right arm.)

### *To Perform the Strength-Training Exercise:*

1. Safety first—always err on the side of a weight that you think will be too light if you're trying an exercise for the first time. Keep your form; movements should be steady and controlled. (If they're not, the weight you're using might be too heavy.) You should have a trainer or a very knowledgeable friend guide you the first few times you engage in strength training.

2. Choose a weight that you can lift no less than 8 times and no more than 12. (The weights you use will slowly increase as you get stronger.)

3. Check for proper body alignment, and then maintain it throughout the exercise.

4. Do two sets of 8 to 12 repetitions of the exercise you have chosen. Doing an exercise once, such as one push-up, is one repetition, or rep. Doing 10 push-ups is 10 reps. A set is a given number of repetitions performed in a row without a break. Therefore, if you have decided to do 2 sets of 10 push-up reps, you will do 10 push-ups, rest briefly, and then do 10 more push-ups.

5. Train to threshold. By this I mean your muscle should be exhausted at the end of the set, and you should feel you couldn't possibly lift the weight one more time. Feeling that maybe you could lift it a few more times if you had to is a sign you're getting stronger, and can slowly increase the weight you're using. (Training to threshold makes your RealAge youngest.)

6. Time your rest intervals. Rest about 45 seconds between sets.

7. Once the exercises become familiar, consider variations. Some (as noted) make the exercise more challenging. Others are just for variety.

8. If your calendar age is over 34, consider taking an aspirin 1 to 2 hours prior to physical activity such as strength training. I urge patients to take a maximum of 2 baby aspirins or 4 ibuprofen or equivalent a day (each with half a glass of warm water before and after taking), and to be careful never to mix aspirin and ibuprofen on the same day. Aspirin makes your arteries and immune system younger and decreases inflammation and pain in your joints.

*Resistance-Training Technique*

Your strength-building exercises can be more effective if you apply the best principles of posture, tempo, and breathing.

## POSTURE

Correct alignment and positioning during exercise and daily activities increase your efficiency and stability and help you avoid injury.

Mom always said, "Stand up straight!" Taken literally, the command can't be done: your spine contains natural (and mandatory) curves. Your neck and lower back curve inward slightly, while your mid- to upper back and your sacrum (tailbone area) curve outward. These curves are needed to absorb shock.

With proper posture, the discs between your vertebrae experience the least stress, enabling support of greater weight without injury. This correct spine alignment is called the set position. To achieve and maintain the set position:

- ■ Pull your shoulder blades back slightly toward each other and down away from your ears.
- ■ Lift your chest up and out.
- ■ Pull your head back just enough to keep it in line with your spine.
- ■ Position your pelvis or hips to create or maintain a natural arch in your lower back. Pull your navel (belly button) in toward your spine without changing your hips (you cannot "tilt" your hips—only your pelvis) and losing the arch in your lower back. Try it now, and practice it every time you do physical activity.

Position a few other body parts to avoid injury:

- ■ Never lock your knees. Keep at least a slight bend in them at all times, and always point your knees in the same direction as your toes (unless your natural leg alignment does not allow it). Your knees should not extend beyond your toes when bending.
- ■ Your elbows should remain slightly bent. Do not lock them.

■ Unless specifically strengthening wrist flexors or extensors, keep your wrists straight and firm.

## TEMPO

Safety should be the prime determinant of how quickly you strength train. The faster the repetition is performed, the more momentum is generated and the greater the risk for injury. Remember, your goal is to maintain perfect technique. Repetitions may last anywhere from 2 to 3 seconds (fast) to 14 seconds (slow). Because muscles adapt to the speed of a contraction, vary the tempo every so often.

Tempo greatly affects the number of repetitions you will be able to perform. If you spend 6 seconds on each repetition, you might reach exhaustion at about the 12-rep mark. On the other hand, you may execute twenty-five 3-second repetitions before fatigue sets in. Your total time under tension for both sets measures roughly the same, but the number of repetitions differs dramatically. Most of the time, use a tempo that exhausts your muscle with that weight at the 8- to 12-repetition mark.

## BREATHING

Don't hold your breath while you lift weights. Resistance training causes blood pressure to rise. If you hold your breath, your blood pressure will rise even more. Exercise physiologists encourage weight lifters to exhale during the exertion phase of each repetition. That's really just a trick to keep you breathing. It also can take your mind off the difficulty of those last tough repetitions. If you are performing faster tempos, breathing in rhythm can lead to hyperventilation. In this case, simply practice continuous, even breathing, and don't worry if your breath patterns aren't synchronized with your exercise rhythm. The timing of your breaths is relatively unimportant, as long as you keep them coming.

Now that you know all that you need to know, let's get started!

### The Exercises

Choose one strengthening exercise to do at threshold from each numbered muscle group. I suggest you start by warming up, and then do your chosen exercises from the odd-numbered groups below, then from the evens, then a second set from the odds, then a second set of evens, and finish with a good set of stretches. Or if you are training every day, do two sets from the odds and two sets from the evens on alternating days. I do evens on even-numbered days, and odds on odd-numbered days, and no strength exercises on the 31st.

These are to help you get started in your weight training. In the beginning, strength training may feel unfamiliar, and you'll need to work carefully to maintain good form. But before you know it, going through your strength-training routine will become second nature. (As you develop skill and want more variety in your exercises, go to our Web site, RealAge.com, for more exercises you can try.)

## EXERCISES FOR YOUR FOUNDATION MUSCLES

### 1. Central Abdominal Muscles

- Basic Abdominal Crunch
- Machine Abdominal Curl

### 2. Lateral Abdominal and Rotator Muscles

- Oblique Figure 4 Crunch
- Trunk Rotation

### 3. Lower Back Muscles

- Prone Back Extension
- Machine Back Extension

### 4. Buttocks, Quadriceps, and Hamstring Muscle Groups

- Basic Squat
- Dumbbell or Barbell Squat
- Machine Squat
- Basic Stationary Lunge
- Dumbbell or Barbell Lunge
- Machine Leg Press

### 5. Upper Back Muscles

- Dumbbell Bent-Over Back Row
- Dumbbell Pull-Over
- Machine Low-Pull Back Row
- Machine Lat Pull-Down

### 6. External Rotators

- Dumbbell Side-Lying External Rotation
- Cable Shoulder External Rotation

### 7. Internal Rotators

- Dumbbell Side-Lying Internal Rotation
- Cable Shoulder Internal Rotation

# 1. CENTRAL ABDOMINAL MUSCLES

## BASIC ABDOMINAL CRUNCH

**Muscle Group(s) Targeted:**

Abdomen (rectus and transverse abdominis)

**Starting Position:**

Lie on your back with your feet braced against the wall or flat on the floor with your knees bent between 60 and 90 degrees. Point the toes slightly outward (at about 11 o'clock and 1 o'clock) if your feet are against the wall, or open your knees slightly if your feet are on the floor. Place your hands behind your head with your elbows pointing directly out to the sides, or cross your arms over your chest.

**Action:**

As you exhale, curl your head and shoulders up and off the floor until your shoulder blades leave the floor and your abdominal muscles are fully contracted. At the same time, pull your navel down toward your spine, flattening and hollowing your abdomen. Slowly roll back down one vertebra at a time to the starting position as you inhale.

**Variation:**

■ You may place your feet higher on the wall in a straight leg position.

**Tips:**

■ Do not pull on your neck with hands. Keep your elbows out wide with your hands just lightly supporting your head.

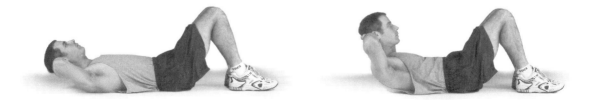

■ It is normal to feel some tension in your neck during this exercise. Your neck muscles are required to lift your head against gravity. If the pain seems to be in your neck bones (vertebrae), however, discontinue this exercise and try one where your head remains on the floor, or try a machine.

■ Your head should stay in line with your spine. Do not point your chin up toward the ceiling or tuck it against your chest.

# MACHINE ABDOMINAL CURL

**Muscle Group(s) Targeted:**

Abdomen (rectus and transverse abdominis)

**Starting Position:**

Adjust the seat height or pad height so the pad sits comfortably on your upper chest or at the front of your shoulders. Grip the handles or rest your arms at your sides. Depending on what kind of machine you are using, either place your feet under the foot pads or on the foot platform. Curl your upper body forward just enough to lift the weight off the stack.

**Action:**

Curl your upper body forward and down without overly bending at the hips. Keep your head in line with your spine, and your navel pulled in toward your spine (this is important for achieving a svelte abdomen). Return to the starting position in a slow, controlled manner.

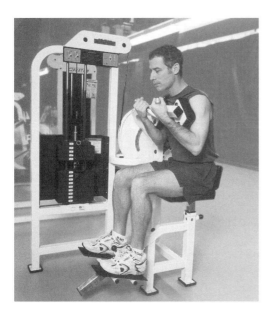
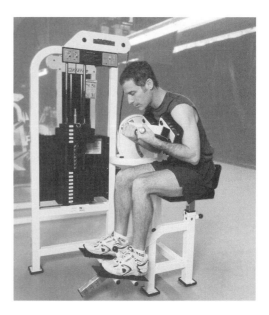

## 2. LATERAL ABDOMINAL AND ROTATOR MUSCLES
## OBLIQUE FIGURE 4 CRUNCH

**Muscle Group(s) Targeted:**

Center and sides of abdomen (rectus abdominis, internal and external obliques)

**Starting Position:**

Lie on your back with your left knee bent and your left foot flat on the floor. Cross your right leg over the left, with your right ankle resting just above the left knee. Place both hands behind your head and your elbows out to the sides.

**Action:**

As you exhale, lift your head and both shoulders up from the floor and twist so that your left armpit moves in a line toward your right knee. Fully contract your abdominals. Inhale as you return toward the starting position. Then switch legs and repeat.

**Variations:**

- Cross your legs more fully, so that one knee rests on the other. This is a more advanced exercise.
- Allow one elbow to remain in contact with the floor. This is a less advanced exercise.

**Tips:**

- Do not allow the elbow to cave in toward your knee. Keep your elbows out wide.
- Keep your head in line with your spine.
- Do not allow the abdominals to relax between repetitions. Keep your head and shoulders slightly off the floor at all times.

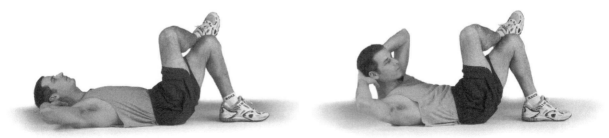

# TRUNK ROTATION

**Muscle Group(s) Targeted:**

Rotators of the spine

**Starting Position:**

Lie on your back with your feet off the floor and your knees bent at 90 degrees. Place your arms, palms down, by your sides, with your head in line with your spine, shoulder blades drawn together and down, a natural arch in your lower back, and navel pulled in toward your spine.

**Action:**

Lower your legs down to one side by rotating your hips without lifting your arms or shoulders off the floor. Do not allow your legs to contact the floor. Slowly pull your legs up and lower them to the opposite side.

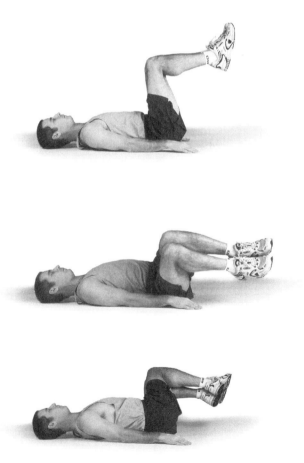

**Variations:**

- Straighten the legs for added resistance (avoid if you have back problems).
- Bend your knees more and bring closer to chest (less challenging).
- For much less resistance, leave your feet on the floor.

**Tip:**

- Keep your upper body stationary throughout the exercise.

## 3. LOWER BACK MUSCLES

## PRONE BACK EXTENSION

**Muscle Group(s) Targeted:**
Back, lower back (erector spinae), buttocks (gluteus maximus), back of thigh (hamstrings)

**Starting Position:**
Lie facedown with your arms at your sides and palms facing the floor, your head in line with your spine, and your shoulder blades drawn together and down. Keep a natural arch in your lower back, and pull your navel in toward your spine.

**Action:**
Lift your head, shoulders, chest, and arms off the floor while keeping your toes in contact with the floor. Maintain your body alignment throughout the exercise. Return to the starting position in a slow, controlled manner.

**Tips:**
- Do not lift your head up too high.
- Do not allow your palms to turn inward toward your body. Keep them facing the floor or turned slightly outward.

**Caution:**
- If you have spondylolysis or spondylolisthesis, do not do this exercise.
- Do not lift your torso to the point of experiencing back pain.

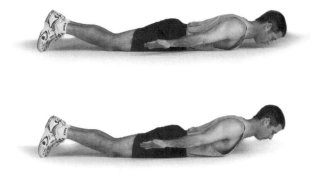

## MACHINE BACK EXTENSION

**Muscle Group(s) Targeted:**

Spine (erector spinae), buttocks (gluteus maximus), back of thigh (hamstrings)

**Starting Position:**

Adjust the back pad so that it is near the center of your back. Sit on the machine with your hips in line with the pivot point (axis) and your feet on the upper or lower foot plate. Keep your head in line with your spine, your shoulder blades drawn together and down, and a natural arch in your lower back. Pull your navel in toward your spine. Your hips should be bent no more than 90 degrees. Press back against the back pad just enough to lift the weight off the stack.

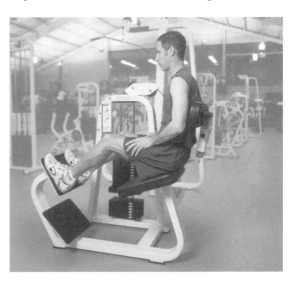

**Action**

Press back against the back pad until you feel that your lower back muscles are fully contracted without causing discomfort. Return to the starting position in a slow, controlled manner.

**Note:**

■ It is easy to confuse back extension and hip extension, and often the two occur simultaneously. True back flexion and extension occur in the spine itself, not in the hips. Although this exercise is called a back extension, it is really more of a hip extension exercise that also involves the lower back muscles and muscles along the spine.

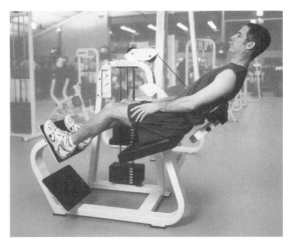

## 4. BUTTOCKS, QUADRICEPS, AND HAMSTRING MUSCLE GROUPS

### BASIC SQUAT, OR DUMBBELL OR BARBELL SQUAT (SAME AS BASIC BUT WITH WEIGHTS)

**Muscle Group(s) Targeted:**

Front of thigh, back of thigh, buttocks (quadriceps, hamstrings, and gluteus)

**Starting Position:**

Stand with your feet about shoulder width apart, knees slightly bent, and toes pointing forward or just slightly out. Hold the dumbbells straight down from your shoulders, or hold the bar just below the base of your neck, slightly above your shoulder blades with your palms facing forward. Keep your focus forward, your chest up, your shoulder blades drawn together and down, your navel pulled in toward your spine, and a natural arch in your lower back. Do not lock your knees.

**Action:**

While keeping your chest lifted, bend your knees, taking your hips back behind you and down toward the floor until your thighs are almost parallel to the floor. Push back up to the starting position.

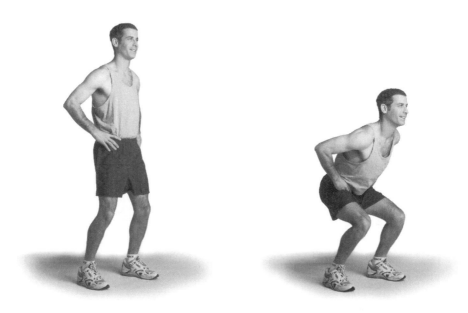

**Tips:**

- Do not allow your knees to extend forward past your toes as you squat.
- Think of taking your hips back behind you rather than straight down.
- Your knees should point in the same direction as your toes, not toward the inside of your feet.
- Keep your heels on the floor.
- Keep your chest lifted and do not lean forward excessively with your upper body.
- You can place a ball between your lower back and a wall and perform the squat against the ball. This is a little tricky to do correctly as your hips need to be moving toward the wall, not forward.

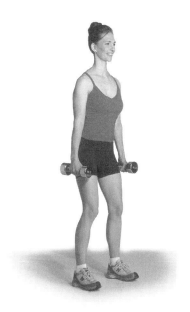

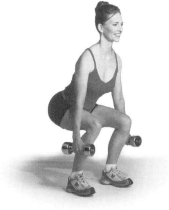

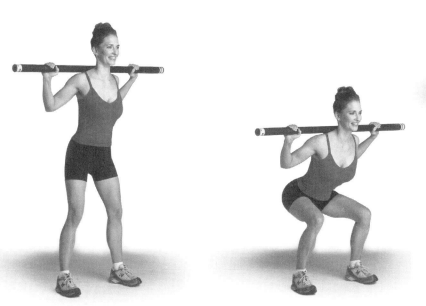

# MACHINE SQUAT

**Muscle Group(s) Targeted:**

Front of thigh, back of thigh, buttocks (quadriceps, hamstrings, and gluteus)

**Starting Position:**

Stand with the bar resting on your upper back (not on the base of your neck), and grip the bar with your hands almost double shoulder width apart. Position yourself so that the weight is over your ankles. Stand with your feet slightly wider than shoulder width, your knees slightly bent, and your legs rotated out about 20 degrees. Bend forward slightly at the hips, keeping the natural arch in your lower back. Keep your focus forward, your chest up, your shoulder blades drawn together and down, and your navel pulled in toward your spine. Do not lock your knees.

**Action:**

While keeping your chest lifted, bend your knees, taking your hips back behind you and down toward the floor until your thighs are almost parallel to the floor. Push back up, keeping the weight centered over your ankles, and return to the starting position.

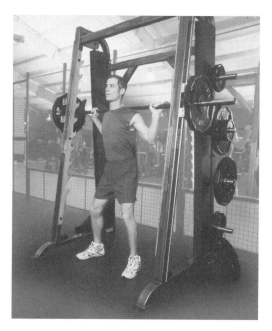 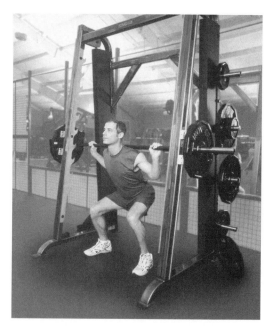

**Tips:**

- Do not allow your knees to extend forward past your toes as you squat.
- Think of taking your hips back behind you rather than straight down.
- Your knees should point in the same direction as your toes, not toward the inside of your feet.
- Keep your heels on the floor.
- Keep your chest lifted and do not lean forward excessively with your upper body.

# BASIC STATIONARY LUNGE, OR DUMBBELL OR BARBELL LUNGE (SAME AS BASIC BUT WITH WEIGHTS)

**Muscle Group(s) Targeted:**

Front of thigh, back of thigh, buttocks (quadriceps, hamstrings, and gluteus)

**Starting Position:**

Stand with your feet at a natural distance apart with one leg in front of the other. Both feet should point directly forward. Center your body weight between both legs. Hold the dumbbells straight down from your shoulders with your palms facing your body, or hold a bar just below the base of your neck, slightly above your shoulder blades, with your palms facing forward. Keep your focus forward, your chest up, your shoulder blades drawn together and down, and your navel pulled in toward your spine. Keep a natural arch in your lower back, and do not lock your knees.

**Action:**

Bend both knees and lower the back knee toward the floor, allowing the back heel to lift off the floor. Stop when the back knee is an inch or two from the floor and your front thigh is roughly parallel to the floor with the knee bent about 90 degrees. Keeping your weight centered or just slightly forward, press back up to the starting position.

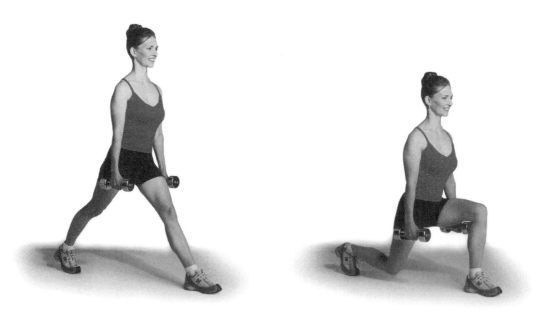

**Variations:**

- Keep your back knee straighter and legs farther apart while lunging.
- Decrease your range of motion and lower yourself only partway down (less challenging).
- Do walking lunges: step forward into each lunge as you alternate sides, or step forward with the same foot each time, bringing the back leg in to meet the front leg between repetitions (more challenging).
- Place the front foot or the back foot on an elevated surface such as a stair or bench.
- Step backward rather than forward into the lunge position.

**Tips:**

- Do not allow your front knee to extend forward past your toes. Lower your weight straight down toward the floor or just slightly forward.
- Keep both feet pointing forward. The tendency is to angle the back foot out slightly, causing a rotational force at the knee during the lunge. This could cause an injury.

# MACHINE LEG PRESS

**Muscle Group(s) Targeted:**
Buttocks (gluteus), back of thigh (hamstrings), front of thigh (quadriceps)

**Starting Position:**
Adjust the distance between the back pad and the foot plate so that your knees are bent no more than 90 degrees when you sit with your back against the pad and your feet on the foot plate. Place your feet about shoulder width apart with your toes pointing directly upward. Keep your sacrum (tailbone area) and mid- to upper back against the back pad. Grasp the handles down at your sides, or allow your hands to rest on your thighs. Keep your shoulder blades drawn together and down, your navel pulled in toward your spine, and a natural arch in your lower back. Press out against the foot plate just enough to lift the weight off the weight stack.

**Action:**
Push the foot plate away from you until your knees are almost straight (not locked). Return to the starting position in a slow, controlled manner.

**Tip:**
   ■ Keep your knees pointing in the same direction as your feet.

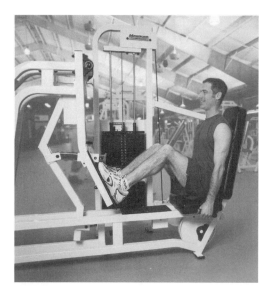 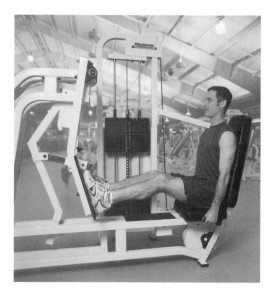

# 5. UPPER BACK MUSCLES

## DUMBBELL BENT-OVER BACK ROW

**Muscle Group(s) Targeted:**

Middle to upper back (latissimus dorsi, teres major, rhomboids, midtrapezius), back of the shoulder (posterior deltoid), front of the upper arm (biceps brachii)

**Starting Position:**

With a dumbbell in one hand, place the opposite hand and knee on a flat bench, so that your spine is straight and roughly parallel to the floor. Allow your arm to hang straight down from your shoulder, with your elbow slightly bent and your wrist straight. Keep your head in line with your spine, your shoulder blades drawn together and down, and a natural arch in your lower back. Do not lock your knees or elbows.

**Action:**

Keeping your elbow and upper arm close to your body, lift the dumbbell in a straight vertical line until it reaches the side of your chest and your upper arm is roughly parallel to the floor. Return to the starting position in a slow, controlled manner.

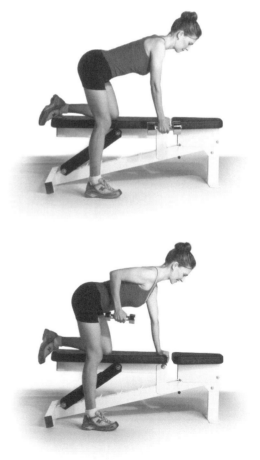

**Tips:**

- Do not allow your back to curve upward or arch excessively.
- Keep your shoulder blades pulled toward each other even between repetitions.
- Do not drop your shoulder toward the floor between repetitions.
- Keep your wrist straight. Do not curl the weight in toward your body.
- Keep your body level, not allowing your torso to twist.
- Lift the weight straight up, not back toward your hip.

# DUMBBELL PULL-OVER

**Muscle Group(s) Targeted:**
Mid- to upper back (latissimus dorsi), back of the shoulder (posterior deltoid)

**Starting Position:**
Position your body faceup, resting your upper back and shoulders (and head if space allows it) across the width of a bench (with your body perpendicular to the bench). You may also lie lengthwise along the bench for extra body support. Keep your feet flat on the floor. Hold the dumbbell securely with both hands (either cupped as with the triceps two-arm overhead extension on page 133 or with both hands gripping the bar) and lift the weight toward the ceiling until your elbows are almost straight and your arms are just past vertical. Keep your head in line with your spine, your shoulder blades drawn together and down, and a natural arch in your lower back. Pull your navel in toward your spine, keep your wrists firm, and do not lock your elbows.

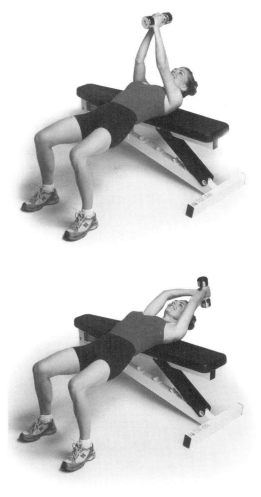

**Action:**
Keeping your elbows in their fixed position (just slightly bent), lower the weight back behind your head until your arms are almost parallel to the floor. Return to the starting position in a slow, controlled manner.

**Tip:**
■ Do not allow your elbows to bend. If you do, this becomes a triceps exercise. Keep your back and hips still, and do not allow your lower back to arch excessively.

**Caution:**
■ Do not drop the weight lower than your head.

# MACHINE LOW-PULL BACK ROW

**Muscle Group(s) Targeted:**

Middle back (latissimus dorsi), front of the upper arm (biceps brachii)

**Starting Position:**

Sit on the bench and grasp the vertical bars on the handle. Put your feet on the foot plates and move back until your knees are bent about 30 degrees and your elbows are just slightly bent. Pull your arms back just enough to lift the weight off the weight stack. Keep your head in line with your spine, your chest up, your shoulder blades drawn together and down, and a natural arch in your lower back. Pull your navel in toward your spine, and keep your wrists firm and straight.

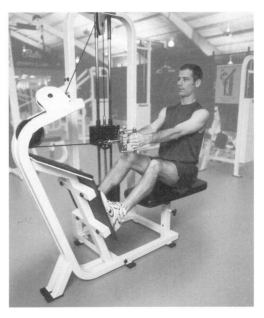

**Action:**

Keeping your arms close to your body, pull the handle toward you until your elbows are at your sides, directly under your shoulders. Return to the starting position in a slow, controlled manner.

**Variation:**

■ This exercise can also be done on other seated row machines that may have different handle angles and may have a chest pad to lean against.

**Tip:**

■ Keep your upper body stationary. Do not allow your torso to lean forward or back as you perform the exercise.

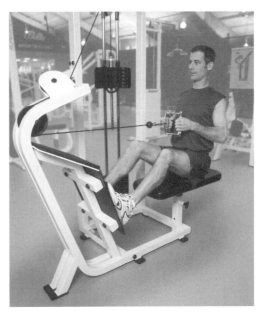

# MACHINE LAT PULL-DOWN

**Muscle Group(s) Targeted:**

Middle to upper back (latissimus dorsi, teres major, rhomboids, trapezius), back of the shoulder (posterior deltoid), front of the upper arm (biceps brachii)

**Starting Position:**

Place your hands on the bar quite a bit wider than shoulder width apart. (Your elbows should create roughly a 90-degree angle when your upper arms are parallel to the floor.) Sit facing the machine with your knees fitting snugly under the pads. Lean your body back about 15 degrees and bend your elbows slightly, just enough to lift the weight off the weight stack. Keep your focus forward, your chest up, your shoulder blades drawn together and down, and a natural arch in your lower back. Pull your navel in toward your spine and keep your wrists firm and straight.

**Action:**

Bend your elbows and pull the bar down until your upper arms are just beyond parallel to the floor. Make sure your elbows stay directly under the bar. Return to the starting position in a slow, controlled manner.

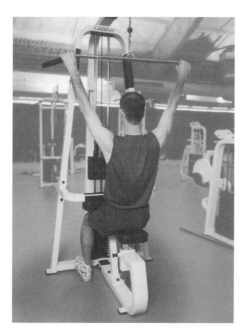 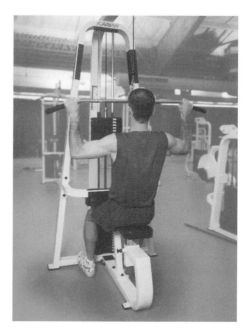

**Variations:**

- Use a wider or a narrower grip.
- Use a narrow, underhand grip so that your palms face you during the exercise.

**Tips:**

- Try to relax your arms and hands and focus on the muscles at the base of your shoulder blades as you perform the exercise.
- Do not pull the bar clear down to your chest. In fact, if the bar is lowered beyond your chin it is probably too far to obtain maximum engagement of your lats.

## 6. EXTERNAL ROTATORS

## DUMBBELL SIDE-LYING EXTERNAL ROTATION

**Muscle Group(s) Targeted:**

Rotator cuff, the external rotators of the shoulder (infraspinatus, teres minor)

**Starting Position:**

Lie on your side on a bench or the floor with a dumbbell in your top hand. Bend the elbow 90 degrees and hold your upper arm against the side of your body with your forearm down across your body. Keep your head in line with your spine, your shoulder blades drawn together, and a natural arch in your lower back. Pull your navel in toward your spine, and keep your wrist firm and straight.

**Action:**

While keeping the upper arm against the side of your body, lift the weight by rotating your shoulder outward. Continue to lift until your forearm is almost perpendicular to the floor. Return to the starting position in a slow, controlled manner.

**Caution:**

■ Do not use a heavy weight with this exercise. Think of it more as a warm-up exercise rather than a strength-building exercise. Stop the exercise before your muscle feels fully fatigued.

■ Some people have more flexibility than others. Do not force your forearm to reach the perpendicular position if it feels at all uncomfortable.

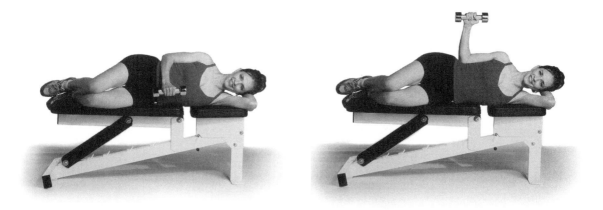

# CABLE SHOULDER EXTERNAL ROTATION

**Muscle Group(s) Targeted:**
External rotators of shoulder (infraspinatus, teres minor)

**Cable Position:**
Set the cable at waist height.

**Starting Position:**
Stand with your side facing the cable machine, your feet shoulder width apart and your knees slightly bent. Grasp the cable handle with the outside hand. Bend that elbow 90 degrees, keeping your upper arm and elbow at your side. Allow the forearm to come across the front of your body with the palm facing you (thumb up). Keep your shoulder blades drawn together and down, and a natural arch in your lower back. Pull your navel in toward your spine, and keep your wrist firm and straight. Step away from the machine until the weight is lifted off the weight stack.

**Action:**
Keeping your elbow and upper arm against the side of your body with your elbow bent 90 degrees, slowly rotate your shoulder outward by bringing your forearm in

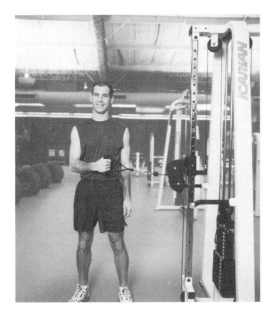 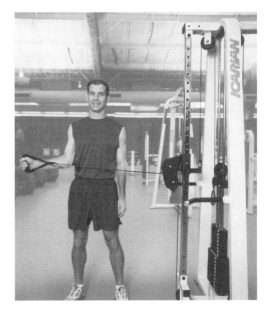

front of you and then out to the side. Your palm faces forward in the end position. Return to the starting position in a slow, controlled manner.

**Tip:**

■ Do not perform this exercise to complete muscle failure. Think of it as a warm-up exercise. Stop as soon as you feel slight fatigue in the shoulder muscles.

**Caution:**

■ Do not use too much resistance with this exercise. The rotators can be easily injured.

# 7. INTERNAL ROTATORS

## DUMBBELL SIDE-LYING INTERNAL ROTATION

**Muscle Group(s) Targeted:**

Rotator cuff, the internal rotator of the shoulder (subscapularis)

**Starting Position:**

Lie on your side on a bench or the floor with a dumbbell in your bottom hand. Place the bottom elbow down at your waist and just in front of your body with your elbow bent 90 degrees and the weight level with the bench or lifted barely off the floor. Keep your head in line with your spine, your shoulder blades drawn together and down, and a natural arch in your lower back. Pull your navel in toward your spine, and keep your wrist firm and straight.

**Action:**

Keeping your bottom elbow on the floor or bench, rotate your shoulder inward, bringing your forearm up and across your waist. Return to the starting position in a slow, controlled manner.

**Caution:**

■ Do not use a heavy weight on this exercise. Think of it more as a warm-up exercise rather than a strength-building exercise. Stop the exercise before your muscle feels fully fatigued.

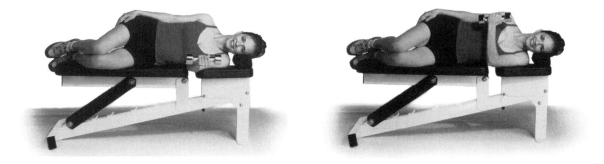

# CABLE SHOULDER INTERNAL ROTATION

**Muscle Group(s) Targeted:**
Rotator of the shoulder (subscapularis)

**Cable Position:**
Set the cable at waist height.

**Starting Position:**
Stand with your side facing the cable machine, feet shoulder width apart and knees slightly bent. Grasp the handle with the hand closest to the machine. Bend your elbow 90 degrees and, keeping the upper arm and elbow close to your body, rotate the shoulder outward, so that your forearm is out to the side and your palm faces forward (thumb up). Step away from the machine until the weight is lifted off the weight stack. Keep your focus forward, your chest up, your shoulder blades drawn together and down, and a natural arch in your lower back. Pull your navel in toward your spine, and keep your wrist firm and straight.

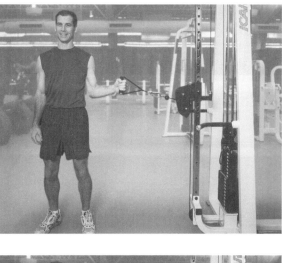

**Action:**
While maintaining your proper alignment, rotate your shoulder inward by bringing your forearm in front of you and across your body. Keep your upper arm and elbow at your side and your wrist firm. Your palm faces your body in this end position. Return to the starting position.

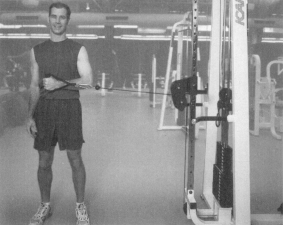

**Caution:**

■ Do not force your forearm out to the side more than is comfortable.

■ Do not use too much resistance with this exercise. The rotators can be easily injured.

### *The Last Lap: Cooldown and Stretching*

We've said it before, but it's one of those things that bears repeating: Too many people view stretching as the optional and dispensable portion of the workout. If you are one of them, change your ways. Immediately.

Every workout session should end with stretching. Stretching gives your mind and body a chance to relax and cool down from your workout.

Stretching improves and/or maintains joint range of motion. Without a normal range of motion in the joints, daily activities become difficult to perform and the risk of musculoskeletal injury increases.

In general, you should perform one stretch for each major muscle group or body part. If several areas feel particularly tight, you may want to choose two or three stretches that target those muscles.

Remember, when you strength train, you are really working those muscles hard. It's extremely important that you take the best possible care of them by following every strength-training session with a cooldown and stretches. The stretches you learned in Chapter 2 should follow your foundation strength-training workout.

After you've done these foundation-strengthening exercises for 30 days, you will be stronger and steadier at your core, and you'll be ready to strengthen and tone the rest of your body. That's what Phase 3 is about.

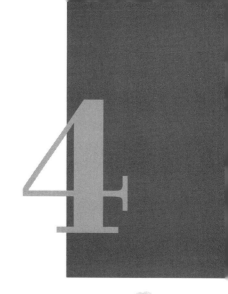

# Phase 3 (Days 61–90): Strengthening Your Non-Foundation Muscles

## Before You Start

By now, you have mastered the art of walking. You genuinely enjoy it and your body starts to ache if you miss even a day. You have also strengthened your foundation muscles. After 30 days of every-other-day strengthening, it takes increasingly heavier weights (whether you use dumbbells or machines) to adhere to the 8- to 12-rule. You may not experience an increase every week, but you can expect to need an increase or two a month for the first 3 months.

If these statements (60 days of walking, 30 days of every-other-day foundation-muscle strengthening) describe you, you are ready to strengthen your non-foundation muscles. If they do not, **do not read any further—do not pass go.** In fact, make a quick U-turn and start from Chapter 1 all over again. Don't be discouraged. Think of this as a second-chance card that allows you to go back to the beginning.

But let's assume you crave the walk and your foundation is stronger than it was.

That means you're ready to take your workout up a notch and start training some of the other muscles in your body. Those muscles are:

### 8. Chest Muscles

This muscle group, which consists of the pectoralis major, runs from your upper arm to your collarbone, breastbone, and ribs. It moves your arms toward the midline of your body and is used in pushing, throwing, and sports that use racquets such as tennis.

### 9. Shoulder Muscles

The shoulder is really a joint, not a muscle group. When we talk of it as a muscle group, we are referring to a group of muscles that act to move or stabilize the shoulder joint. These include the deltoid, which cups the front, top, and back of your shoulder, and the rotator cuff, which consists of four muscles that rotate the shoulder and stabilize your upper arm in the shoulder socket. Almost every activity you do with your arms requires you to use some combination of the deltoid and rotator cuff muscles. The moment you start to lift your arm, you are using these muscles. It is important to keep a balance of strength and flexibility in these muscles in order to avoid debilitating injuries.

### 10. Biceps

Your biceps muscle is located on the front of your upper arm between your shoulder and your elbow. This is the Popeye the Sailor muscle, the one that bulges when someone bends an elbow to "make a muscle." The biceps, along with a couple of other muscles, serves primarily to bend your elbow.

### 11. Triceps

Your triceps muscle, as the name implies, has three parts. It is found on the back of your upper arm, just opposite your biceps. It performs the opposite action of the biceps: It straightens your elbow against resistance. You use your triceps whenever you push something away from you, lift something over your head, or push yourself up by your arms from a seated position, when, for example, you get up from an armchair.

## 12. Forearms

Your forearm has four main muscle groups. One is located on the topside of your forearm. These muscles keep your hands steady for activities such as typing or playing the piano. On the opposite side of your forearm, on the underside of your arm, are the wrist flexors. They can curl your hands toward you when your palms are facing up, such as when you are carrying bags of groceries. The last groups are located deeper in the forearm, and they allow you to rotate your forearm, a movement often called supination and pronation. The exercises we will describe are primarily for the topside of your forearm. (The underside of your forearm is strengthened in many of the biceps exercises.)

At this stage of the game, there are some rules to follow:

1. Choose one exercise from each of the muscle groups. You can vary the exercise for any one muscle group you choose, but we suggest you master one from each group first. Warm up for each exercise with a lighter weight.
2. Exercise each muscle group 3 times a week, preferably every other day, and do not exercise the same muscle group on consecutive days.
3. Use the 8- to 12-repetition rule. If you cannot lift it with perfect form 8 times, choose a lighter weight; if you can lift it more than 12 times with perfect form and without feeling totally fatigued, choose a heavier weight. Perform 2 sets of each exercise.
4. Exercise the muscle groups in the order they are listed.
5. Stretch each muscle you have exercised at the end of your workout.

### *The Exercises to Strengthen the Non-Foundation Muscles*

### 8. Chest Muscles

- Basic Push-Up
- Dumbbell or Barbell Chest Press
- Dumbbell Chest Fly

- Machine Chest Press
- Machine Chest Fly
- Machine Cable Crossovers

## 9. Shoulder Muscles

- Dumbbell Side Raise
- Dumbbell Front Raise
- Dumbbell Arnold Press
- Machine Side Raise
- Machine Overhead Press

## 10. Biceps

- Dumbbell or Barbell Biceps Curl
- Dumbbell Concentration Curl
- Machine Biceps Preacher Curl
- Cable Biceps Curl

## 11. Triceps

- Triceps Dip
- Dumbbell One-Arm Overhead Extension
- Dumbbell Two-Arm Overhead Extension
- Dumbbell Lying Two-Arm Triceps Extension
- Dumbbell Triceps Kick-Back
- Gravity-Assisted Triceps Dip with Machine
- Machine Triceps Extension
- Cable Triceps Press-Down
- Reverse Grip Triceps Pull-Down
- Cable Triceps Overhead Press-Out

## 12. Forearms

- Dumbbell or Barbell Forearm (Reverse) Curl
- Tubing Forearm (Reverse) Curl

# 8. CHEST MUSCLES

## BASIC PUSH-UP

**Muscle Group(s) Targeted:**

Chest, front of the shoulder, back of the upper arm (pectoralis major and minor, anterior deltoid, triceps)

**Starting Position:**

Place your hands on the floor slightly wider than shoulder width. Extend your legs and body so that only your toes touch the floor, and so that your head, spine, and legs form a straight line. Keep your elbows slightly bent, your head in line with your spine, your shoulder blades drawn together and down, and a natural arch in your lower back. Pull your navel in toward your spine.

**Action:**

Keeping your head, back, and legs in a straight line by tightening your abdominal muscles, lower your body toward the floor until your upper arms are roughly parallel to the floor (approximately 90-degree bend at your elbows). Keep your elbows directly over your hands. Press your body back up to the starting position.

**Variations:**

■ For a less challenging push-up, you can rest your knees on the floor or do the push-up against a wall or against an elevated object, such as a tabletop.

■ For a more challenging push-up, elevate your feet, or lift one leg, or have one arm behind your back.

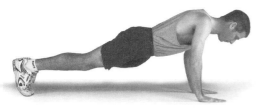 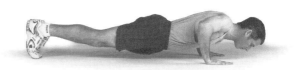

**Tips:**

■ Place your hands and arms in line with your chest, not up toward your face or back toward your ribs.

■ Do not allow your back or hips to sag or lift up during the exercise.

**Caution:**

■ Do not lock your knees or elbows.

# DUMBBELL OR BARBELL CHEST PRESS

**Muscle Group(s) Targeted:**

Chest, front of the shoulder, back of the upper arm (pectoralis major and minor, anterior deltoid, triceps)

**Starting Position:**

Lie on your back on a flat bench with your knees bent and feet flat on the floor. If it is more comfortable, place your feet on the bench instead of on the floor. Hold the dumbbells straight up from your shoulders with your elbows slightly bent and palms forward, or grip the barbell slightly wider than shoulder width. Your arms should be roughly perpendicular to the floor.

**Action:**

Bend your elbows out to the sides and lower the weight until your elbows are bent about 90 degrees and your upper arms are parallel to the floor. The dumbbells should remain directly over your elbows. Press the weights back up to the starting position by bringing your arms up and toward each other, with your shoulder blades drawn together and a natural but not excessive arch in your lower back. Pull your navel in toward your spine, and keep your wrists firm.

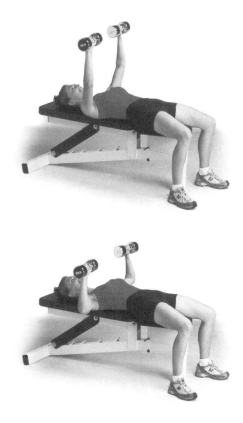

**Tips:**

■ Do not lift your hips off the bench.

■ Keep your wrists firm, straight, and directly over your elbows.

**Caution:**

■ Do not lower your elbows below the height of the bench. It is inefficient in working your chest muscles and could cause shoulder injury.

■ Never lock your elbows at the top of the motion.

# DUMBBELL CHEST FLY

**Muscle Group(s) Targeted:**
Chest, front of the shoulder (pectoralis major and minor, shoulder girdle muscles)

**Starting Position:**
Lie on your back on a flat bench or the floor with your knees bent and feet flat on the floor. If it is more comfortable, place your feet up on the bench instead of on the floor. Hold the dumbbells straight up from your shoulders with your palms facing each other and your elbows slightly bent. Keep your shoulder blades drawn together, your wrists firm, and a natural arch in your lower back. Pull your navel in toward your spine.

**Action:**
Keeping your elbows slightly bent, lower the weights down and out to the sides until your elbows are even with your shoulders. Return to the starting position by bringing the arms up and toward each other.

**Tips:**
■ Do not lock your elbows.
■ Do not lift your hips off the bench or allow your back to arch excessively.
■ Do not lower your arms beneath the level of your shoulders. In the open position, you should be able to see both hands in your peripheral vision. If you cannot, your arms are down too far.

**Caution:**
■ Keep the weight manageable on this exercise. Do not try to use as much weight as you use for the chest press.

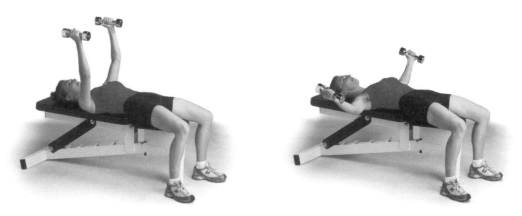

# MACHINE CHEST PRESS

**Muscle Group(s) Targeted:**

Chest, front of the shoulder, back of the upper arm (pectoralis major and minor, anterior deltoid, triceps)

**Starting Position:**

Adjust the seat height so that your arms are roughly parallel to the floor when you hold on to the horizontal handles. Sit with your sacrum, mid- to upper back, and head against the bench, with your feet flat on the floor or on the footrests. Press your arms forward until the weight is fully in your possession and your upper arms are straight out to the sides of your body with your elbows bent 90 degrees. Keep your chest up, your shoulder blades drawn together and down, your wrists firm and straight, and a natural arch in your lower back. Pull your navel in toward your spine.

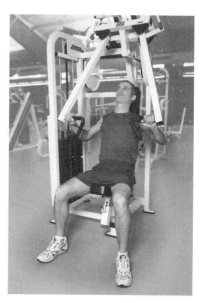

**Action:**

Press your arms forward until they are straight but not locked. Return to the starting position in a slow, controlled manner.

**Variation:**

■ You may use the vertical handles.

**Tip:**

■ Do not allow your elbows to extend behind your shoulders between repetitions.

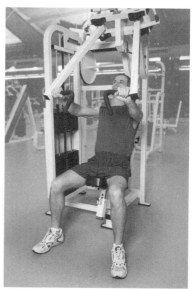

# MACHINE CHEST FLY

**Muscle Group(s) Targeted:**
Chest, front of the shoulder (pectoralis major and minor, shoulder girdle muscles)

**Starting Position:**
Adjust the seat height so that your arms are at chest level when you grasp the handles or when you are using other machines place your inner arms against the pads. Keep a slight bend in your elbows, and stay in contact with the back pad. Your arms should be slightly in front of your shoulders with your hands visible in your peripheral vision. Keep your chest up, your shoulder blades drawn together and down, and a natural arch in your lower back. Pull your navel in toward your spine. Keep your wrists firm and straight, and do not lock your elbows. Press your arms forward just enough to lift the weight off the weight stack.

**Action:**
Pull your arms toward each other until your hands are just narrower than shoulder width. Return to the starting position in a slow, controlled manner.

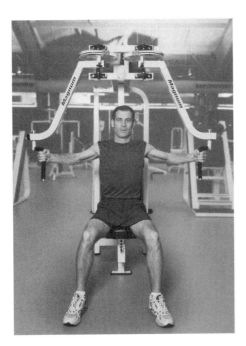 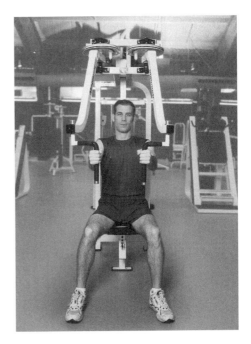

**Variation:**

■ You may use either the vertical or horizontal handles. Generally use the vertical handles when working against higher resistances.

**Caution:**

■ Use a different chest exercise if you experience forearm pain or discomfort near the crease of your elbows.

# MACHINE CABLE CROSSOVERS

**Muscle Group(s) Targeted:**

Chest, front of the shoulder (pectoralis major and minor, shoulder girdle muscles)

**Starting Position:**

Grasp both handles from the tops of the pulleys and stand centered between the cable machines. Bend forward from your hips about 45 degrees, keeping your knees slightly bent and maintaining the natural arch in your lower back. Pull your arms toward each other and toward the floor until your hands are just narrower than shoulder width, with your palms facing each other and your elbows slightly bent. Keep your head in line with your spine, your shoulder blades drawn together, your wrists firm and straight, your knees slightly bent, and a natural arch in your lower back. Pull your navel in toward your spine.

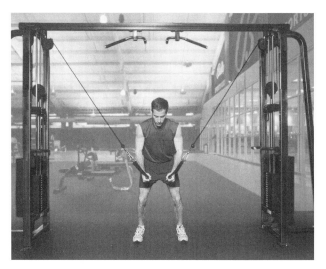

**Action:**

Keeping your body stationary, slowly move your arms up and out to the sides until they are almost parallel to the floor. Press back down to the starting position.

**Variation:**

■ By changing the degree to which you are bent for-

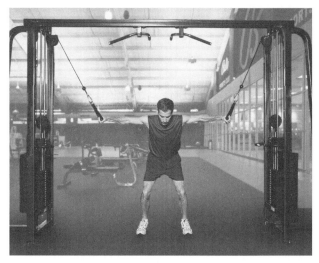

ward, you can adjust the angle of resistance to focus on different parts of your chest.

**Caution:**

■ Do not allow your elbows to extend behind your back, because this decreases the pectoral involvement and could cause shoulder injury.

■ If you have back problems, choose a different chest exercise.

# 9. SHOULDER MUSCLES
## DUMBBELL SIDE RAISE

**Muscle Group(s) Targeted:**

Front and top of the shoulder, top of the shoulder blade (deltoid and shoulder girdle muscles)

**Starting Position:**

Stand with your feet about shoulder width apart and with your knees slightly bent. Lean forward slightly from the hips and let your arms hang straight down with your elbows slightly bent and palms facing each other. Lift your arms out to the sides just a few inches from your thighs to begin engaging your shoulder muscles. Keep your focus forward, your chest up, your shoulder blades drawn together and down, and a natural arch in your lower back. Pull your navel in toward your spine. Keep your wrists firm and straight, and do not lock your elbows or knees.

**Action:**

Raise your arms up and out to your sides until your arms are almost parallel to the floor and your hands are slightly in front of your shoulders, in your peripheral vision.

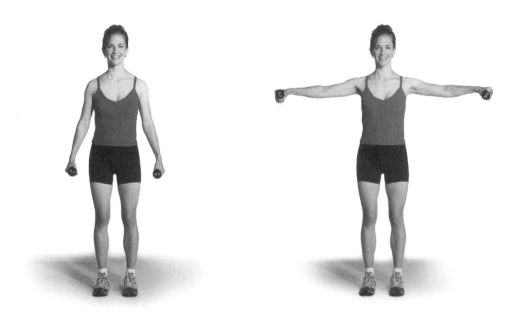

Keep your wrists straight and elbows slightly bent. Return to the starting position in a slow, controlled manner.

**Variations:**

- Use one arm at a time, either alternating arms with each repetition or completing an entire set with one arm before changing to the other arm.
- Perform the exercise with your elbows bent 90 degrees (your upper arm still performs the same motion as described).
- Perform in a seated position.

**Tip:**

- You may decrease your range of motion and not lift the arms as high if you experience shoulder discomfort.

**Caution:**

- The shoulder is not particularly strong in the abducted position. Use light weights for this exercise and discontinue it if shoulder pain develops.
- Do not lift your arms higher than your shoulders.

# DUMBBELL FRONT RAISE

**Muscle Group(s) Targeted:**
Front of the shoulder, chest (deltoid, shoulder girdle, pectoralis major)

**Starting Position:**
Stand with your feet about shoulder width apart and your knees slightly bent. Hold the dumbbells a few inches in front of your thighs with your elbows slightly bent and your palms facing each other. Keep your focus forward, your chest up, your shoulder blades drawn together and down, and a natural arch in your lower back. Pull your navel in toward your spine. Keep your wrists firm, and do not lock your elbows or knees.

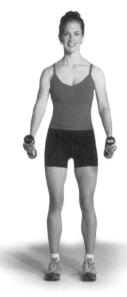

**Action:**
Lift your arms up in front of you and slightly out until they are roughly at shoulder height and slightly wider than shoulder width. Keep your elbows slightly bent. Lower your arms to the starting position in a slow, controlled manner.

**Variations:**
- Use one arm at a time, alternating arms with each repetition or completing an entire set with one arm before changing to the other arm.
- You may also perform the exercise with your palms facing your thighs in the start position and the floor in the end position.

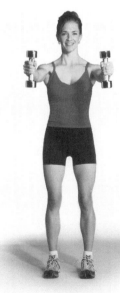

**Tip:**
- Do not allow your body to sway or shift forward or backward.

**Caution:**
- When selecting the weight for this exercise, go lighter rather than heavier, and discontinue the exercise if shoulder pain develops.

# DUMBBELL ARNOLD PRESS

**Muscle Group(s) Targeted:**
Front and top of the shoulder, back of the upper arm (deltoid, shoulder girdle, triceps)

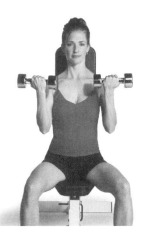

**Starting Position:**
Sit on a bench or chair with or without back support, and rest your feet flat on the floor. Hold the dumbbells in front of your shoulders with your palms facing your shoulders and your elbows pointed down. Your forearms should be perpendicular to the floor, and the dumbbells should be directly above your elbows. Keep your focus forward, your shoulder blades drawn together and down, and a natural arch in your lower back. Pull your navel in toward your spine.

**Action:**
Press the weights upward as you rotate your arms, so that your palms face forward when your arms are extended over your head. Keep the weights aligned directly above your elbows throughout the movement. Return to the starting position in a slow, controlled manner.

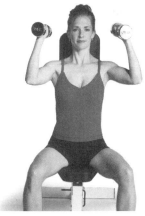

**Variations:**
- Do the exercise in a standing position (more challenging to keep proper alignment).
- Do one arm at a time, either alternating arms with each repetition or completing an entire set with one arm before switching to the other arm.

**Tips:**
- Keep your back erect, and do not allow any torso movement.
- Keep your wrists firm and straight.
- Do not lock your elbows at the top of the movement.

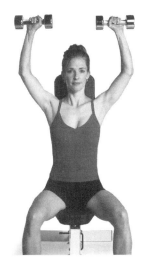

**Caution:**

- Stop this exercise if you experience any popping, clicking, or discomfort.
- If you suffer from impingement in your shoulder joint, try using a bench with back support and angle it back slightly, so that you are lifting the weight slightly in front of your shoulders rather than directly over your head. If you are still experiencing discomfort, stop the exercise.

# MACHINE SIDE RAISE

**Muscle Group(s) Targeted:**

Front and top of the shoulder, top of the shoulder blade (deltoid, shoulder girdle)

**Starting Position:**

Adjust the seat height so that the arm pads rest on the sides of your arms just above your elbows, with the upper arms down at your sides and your forearms parallel to the floor (elbows bent 90 degrees). Your shoulders should be aligned with the pivot point of the machine. Grasp the handles with your palms facing each other. Keep your focus forward, your shoulder blades drawn together and down, and a natural arch in your lower back. Pull your navel in toward your spine and raise your arms out to the sides just enough to lift the weight off the weight stack.

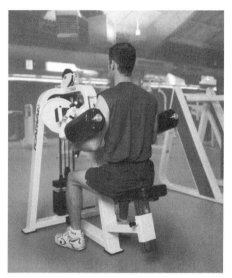

**Action:**

Raise your arms out to the sides until they are about parallel to the floor and palms are facing down. Return to the starting position in a slow, controlled manner.

**Tip:**

■ Keep your shoulders down as you lift your arms.

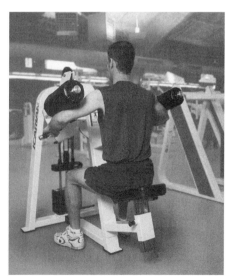

# MACHINE OVERHEAD PRESS

**Muscle Group(s) Targeted:**

Front and top of the shoulder, back of the upper arms (deltoid, triceps, shoulder girdle)

**Starting Position:**

Adjust the seat height so that your hands are a few inches higher than your shoulders and your elbows are bent a little more than 90 degrees when you grasp the handles. You may either position your palms forward or facing each other. Your hands should be toward the front of your shoulders. Keep your focus forward, your shoulder blades drawn together and down, your wrists firm and straight, and a natural arch in your lower back. Pull your navel in toward your spine. Press your arms upward enough to lift the weight off the weight stack.

**Action:**

Press your arms up until your elbows are almost straight. Return to the starting position in a slow, controlled manner.

**Caution:**

- ■ Your arms or hands should never be behind your shoulders. This places your shoulders at risk in an overly externally rotated position.
- ■ Stop this exercise if you experience any popping, clicking, or discomfort.

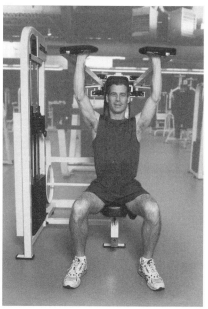

# 10. BICEPS

## DUMBBELL OR BARBELL BICEPS CURL

**Muscle Group(s) Targeted:**
Front of the upper arm, forearm (biceps, brachioradialis)

**Starting Position:**
Stand with your feet approximately shoulder width apart and your knees slightly bent. Hold the dumbbells at your sides with your palms facing forward and your elbows slightly bent, or hold the barbell just in front of your thighs with your hands shoulder width apart and your palms facing forward. Keep your focus forward, your chest up, your shoulder blades drawn together and down, your wrists firm and straight, and a natural arch in your lower back. Pull your navel in toward your spine and do not lock your elbows or knees.

**Action:**
Bend your elbows and bring your hands up toward your shoulders while keeping your elbows down at your sides, directly under your shoulders. Return to the starting position.

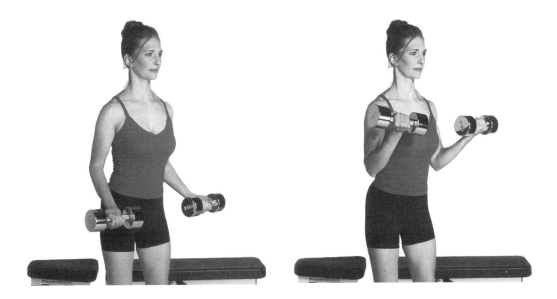

**Variations:**

- You may do a dumbbell biceps curl while seated on a bench, ball, or stool.
- With the dumbbell curl, you may start with your palms facing each other and rotate your palms to face your shoulders as you lift the weights.
- With the dumbbell curl, you may do one arm at a time, alternating arms with each repetition or performing all repetitions with one arm first and then the other.

**Tips:**

- Keep your upper arms stationary. Do not allow any shoulder movement.
- Keep your trunk stationary. Do not allow any back-and-forth motion.

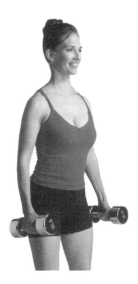
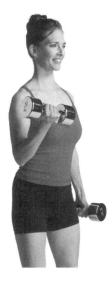

# DUMBBELL CONCENTRATION CURL

**Muscle Group(s) Targeted:**

Front of the upper arm, forearm (biceps, brachioradialis)

**Starting Position:**

Sit on a bench, chair, or ball with your legs apart and feet flat on the floor. With a weight in one hand, lean forward and rest the back of that elbow or upper arm against your inner thigh with your palm facing the opposite foot. Keep your elbow slightly bent, your head in line with your spine, your shoulder blades drawn together and down, and as much as possible, a natural arch in your lower back. Pull your navel in toward your spine. Keep your wrist firm, and do not lock your elbow. Place your other hand or forearm on top of your other thigh to support yourself.

**Action:**

Keeping your upper arm stationary, lift the dumbbell up toward your shoulder until your elbow is bent more than 90 degrees but the weight is still at least 6 inches from your shoulder. Return to the starting position in a slow, controlled manner.

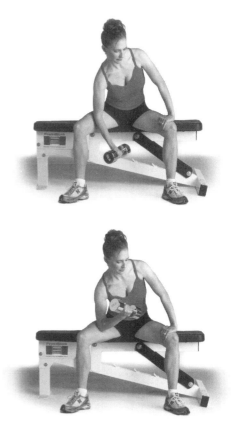

**Variation:**

■ Start with your palm facing inward toward your body. (Your forearm is turned inward as opposed to the original exercise description.)

**Tips:**

■ Do not allow any upper arm or shoulder movement.

■ Support your torso weight with your arm and not with your back.

**Caution:**

■ Choose a different biceps exercise if you experience any back discomfort.

# MACHINE BICEPS PREACHER CURL

**Muscle Group(s) Targeted:**
Front of the upper arm, forearm (biceps, brachioradialis)

**Starting Position:**
Adjust the seat height so your arms are parallel to the floor while resting straight in front of you on the arm pads. Move your body forward or back so your elbows are in line with the axis or pivot point of the machine. Keep your chest up, your shoulder blades drawn together and down, your wrists firm and straight, and a natural arch in your lower back. Pull your navel in toward your spine, and do not lock your elbows. With your palms facing up, grasp the handles. Bend your elbows just enough to lift the weights off the weight stack.

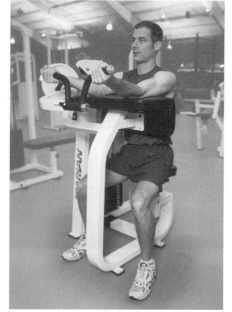

**Action:**
Keeping your shoulders and upper arms still, pull your hands up and toward you until your elbows are bent a little more than 90 degrees. Return to the starting position in a slow, controlled manner.

**Tip:**
■ Do not allow your shoulders to roll forward.

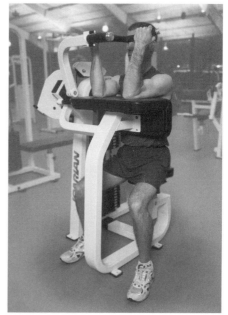

# CABLE BICEPS CURL

**Muscle Group(s) Targeted:**

Front of the upper arm, forearm (biceps, brachioradialis)

**Starting Position:**

Attach a bar to the end of the cable. Stand facing the cable unit with your feet shoulder width apart and knees slightly bent. Grasp the bar with your palms facing forward and slightly more than shoulder width apart, with your arms down at your sides. Keep your focus forward, your chest up, your shoulder blades drawn together and down, your wrists firm and straight, and a natural arch in your lower back. Pull your navel in toward your spine, and do not lock your elbows or knees. Bend your elbows slightly and stand back far enough that the weight is lifted off the stack.

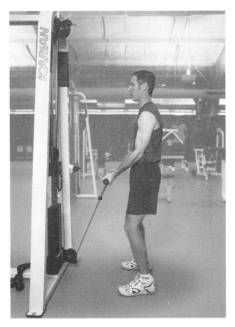

**Action:**

Hinging at your elbows, lift the bar as close to your shoulders as possible without bending your wrists or moving your upper arms. Return to the starting position in a slow, controlled manner.

**Tips:**

■ Do not lean back as you lift the bar.
■ Keep your shoulders and upper arms still to maximize bicep involvement.

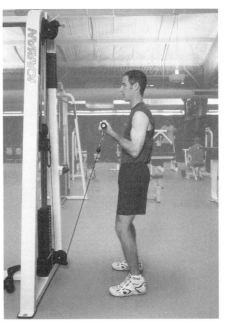

# 11. TRICEPS

## TRICEPS DIP

**Muscle Group(s) Targeted:**
Back of the upper arm (triceps)

**Starting Position:**
Facing away from a secure object such as a bench or desk, place your hands shoulder width apart and grasp the edge of the supporting surface. Place your feet on the floor in front of you, so your knees are bent between 10 and 90 degrees (the more bent, the easier the exercise). Your hands and elbows should be directly under your shoulders, with your elbows slightly bent. Keep your focus forward, your chest up, your shoulder blades drawn together and down, and, as much as possible, a natural arch in your lower back. Pull your navel in toward your spine.

**Action:**
Lower your body toward the floor until your elbows are bent about 90 degrees (less if you experience discomfort). Press down with your arms to raise yourself back to the starting position.

**Variations:**
- For lighter resistance, place your feet flat on the floor close to the bench.
- For heavier resistance, extend your legs and move your feet farther from the bench.
- Lift one leg off the floor and cross it over the other leg or hold it straight out.
- Elevate both feet using some sort of platform. You can also place weights on your hips or thighs in this position to add resistance.

**Tip:**
- You can use your legs as much or as little as you need to help you press back up to the starting position.

**Caution:**

■ Do not bend your elbows more than 90 degrees, because this can stretch the supporting structures of your shoulder.

■ Stop the exercise if you experience shoulder or elbow pain.

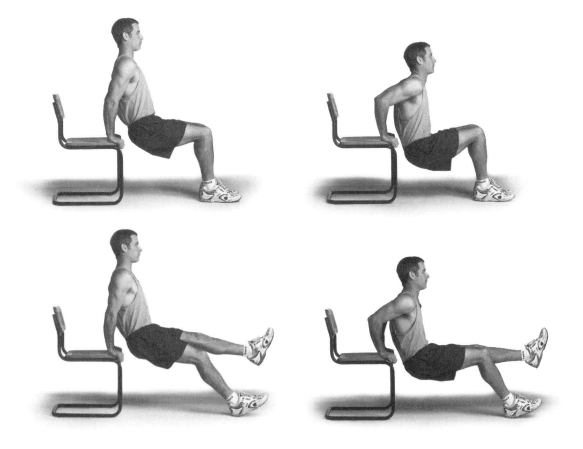

# DUMBBELL ONE-ARM OVERHEAD EXTENSION

**Muscle Group(s) Targeted:**

Back of the upper arm (triceps)

**Starting Position:**

Sit on a bench or chair with a weight in one hand. Straighten your arm up above your head (with your elbow slightly bent) so that your upper arm is close to your ear and your elbow is facing forward or out to the side. Keep your head in line with your spine, your shoulder blades drawn together, your wrist firm and straight, and a natural arch in your lower back. Do not lock your elbow.

**Action:**

Lower the weight behind your head, keeping your elbow high and the upper arm stationary. Press the weight back up to return to the starting position.

**Tip:**

■ Keep your elbow high, never allowing your upper arm to move away from the side of your head.

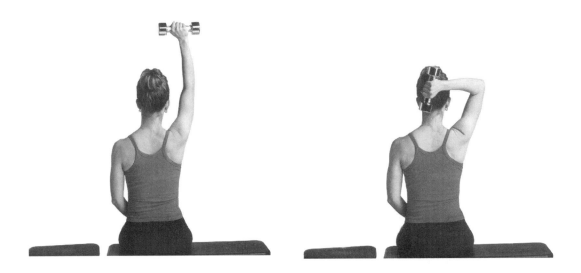

# DUMBBELL TWO-ARM OVERHEAD EXTENSION

**Muscle Group(s) Targeted:**

Back of the upper arm (triceps)

**Starting Position:**

Cup the end of a dumbbell with both hands, so that your eight fingers point behind you, your thumbs are forward, and your hands form a cup on which one end of the weight rests. (You may hold the handle securely with both hands instead if this is more comfortable.) Extend your arms over your head with your elbows slightly bent. Keep your head in line with your spine, your shoulder blades drawn together and down, your wrists firm, and a natural arch in your lower back. Pull your navel in toward your spine, and do not lock your elbows.

**Action:**

Keep your upper arms roughly perpendicular to the floor as you lower the weight behind your head until your elbows are bent approximately 90 degrees. Press the weight back up to return to the starting position.

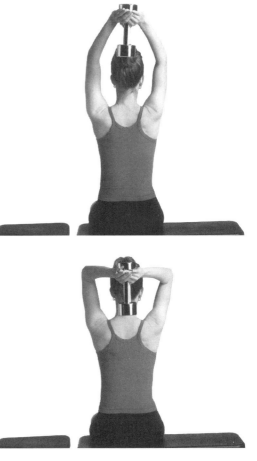

**Tip:**

■ Do not allow much movement of your upper arms as you lower the weight. Your elbows should remain high and fairly close to your head.

**Caution:**

■ This exercise takes a certain degree of shoulder flexibility. If you feel like you must crane your head forward or slouch in order to have the weight miss your head, or if you experience shoulder discomfort, choose a different exercise.

■ Keep the weight far enough from your head that the weight does not hit your head.

# DUMBBELL LYING TWO-ARM TRICEPS EXTENSION

**Muscle Group(s) Targeted:**
Back of the upper arm (triceps)

**Starting Position:**
Lie on your back on the floor or a bench with your feet flat on the floor. Press the dumbbells straight up from your shoulders with your palms facing each other and your elbows slightly bent. Keep your head in line with your spine, your shoulder blades drawn together and down, a natural arch in your lower back, and your wrists firm and straight. Pull your navel in toward your spine, and do not lock your elbows. Your arms should be roughly perpendicular to the floor.

**Action:**
Keeping your upper arms stationary, bend your elbows and lower the weights to either side of your head until your elbows are bent about 90 degrees. Press the weights back up to return to the starting position.

**Variation:**
■ You may do the exercise with one arm and place the opposite hand on the back of the upper arm to give some stability and support.

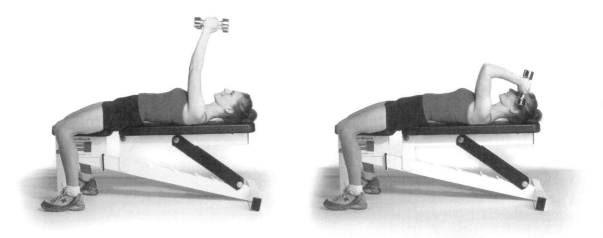

**Tips:**

- If you have an excessive arch in your lower back when lying on a bench with your feet on the floor, try placing your feet on elevated blocks or up on the bench with your knees bent.
- Do not allow your upper arms to move down or out to the sides. Keep your elbows up and your upper arms still.
- If you do not feel this working your triceps, try moving your arms slightly past the vertical position, so that your upper arms are a little closer to your head.

**Caution:**

- This exercise is called the skull crusher by some for obvious reasons. It is most safely done with a spotter, at least until you have mastered the motion.
- Stop this exercise if you feel pain or burning in your elbows.

# DUMBBELL TRICEPS KICK-BACK

**Muscle Group(s) Targeted:**
Back of the upper arm (triceps)

**Starting Position:**
With a dumbbell in one hand, place the opposite hand and knee on a flat bench so your spine is straight and roughly parallel to the floor. Keep your head in line with your spine, your shoulder blades drawn together and down, a natural arch in your lower back, and your wrist firm and straight. Pull your navel in toward your spine, and do not lock your elbows or knees. Bend your elbow about 80 degrees, so your upper arm is parallel to the floor and your forearm is just short of vertical, with your palm facing in.

**Action:**
Keeping your upper arm stationary, extend the dumbbell back until your arm is straight and roughly parallel to the floor. Return to the starting position in a slow, controlled manner.

**Tip:**

■ Keep your wrist firm and upper arm still. Do not allow any shoulder movement.

**Caution:**

■ Switch to a different triceps exercise if you experience shoulder or elbow pain with this exercise.

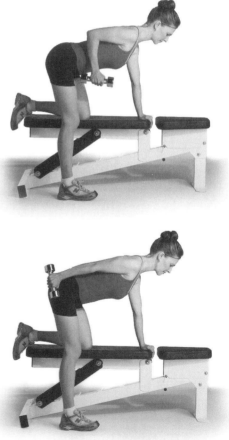

# GRAVITY-ASSISTED TRICEPS DIP WITH MACHINE

**Muscle Group(s) Targeted:**

Back of the upper arm (triceps)

**Starting Position:**

While keeping at least one foot on an immobile foot support, rotate the dip bars (closer together or apart) so that your hands are directly under your shoulders when you grasp the bars, palms facing your body. Place your knees on the mobile support pad with your arms down at your sides and elbows slightly bent. Keep your focus forward, your shoulder blades drawn together and down, a natural arch in your lower back, and your wrists firm and straight. Pull your navel in toward your spine, and do not lock your elbows.

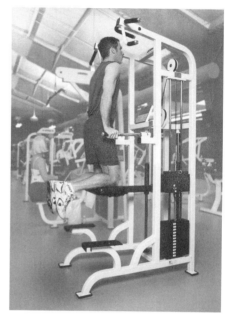

**Action:**

Lower your body toward the floor until your elbows are bent about 90 degrees (or less if you experience any discomfort). Press down with your arms to raise yourself back to the starting position.

**Caution:**

■ Do not bend your elbows more than 90 degrees, because this can strain your shoulders' supporting structures.

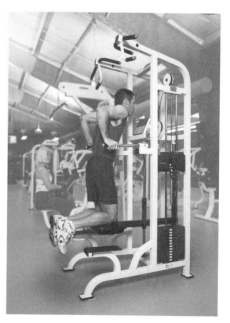

# MACHINE TRICEPS EXTENSION

**Muscle Group(s) Targeted:**

Back of the upper arm (triceps)

**Starting Position:**

Adjust the seat height so that your elbows reach the end of the angled arm pad when you lean forward against the chest pad. Lower the thigh pads until they contact your thighs. Bring the handles toward your ears and grip them with your palms facing each other. Keep your focus forward, your shoulder blades drawn together and down, a natural arch in your lower back, and your wrists firm and straight. Pull your navel in toward your spine. Press forward with your hands just enough to lift the weight off the stack.

**Action:**

Press your forearms forward and down until your elbows are straight. Return to the starting position in a slow, controlled manner.

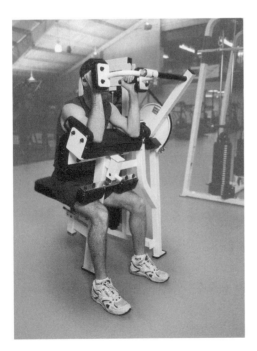 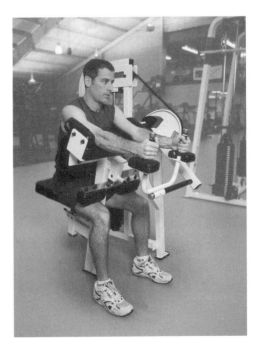

# CABLE TRICEPS PRESS-DOWN

**Muscle Group(s) Targeted:**

Back of the upper arm (triceps)

**Starting Position:**

Attach a bar or a rope handle to the end of the cable. Stand facing the cable unit with your feet a comfortable distance apart and your knees slightly bent. Lean forward slightly from your hips. Grasp the bar with an overhand grip, with your hands shoulder width apart. Bend your elbows a little more than 90 degrees and position them directly under your shoulders so that your upper arms are roughly perpendicular to the floor, and close to your sides. Keep your focus forward, your shoulder blades drawn together and down, a natural arch in your lower back, and your wrists firm and straight. Pull your navel in toward your spine. Press down just enough to lift the weight slightly off the weight stack.

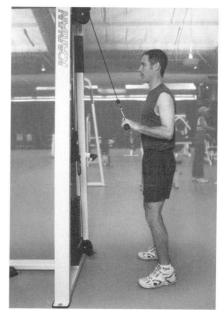

**Action:**

Keeping your upper arms stationary, press the bar down to your thighs. Return to the starting position in a slow, controlled manner.

**Tip:**

■ Do not allow any torso or upper arm movement.

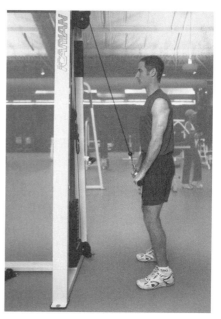

# REVERSE GRIP TRICEPS PULL-DOWN

**Muscle Group(s) Targeted:**
Back of the upper arm (triceps)

**Starting Position:**
Attach a bar to the end of the cable from a high pulley position. Stand facing the cable unit with your feet a comfortable distance apart and your knees slightly bent. With both hands, grasp the bar with an underhand grip, with your hands shoulder width apart. Keep your focus forward, your shoulder blades drawn together and down, a natural arch in your lower back, and your wrists firm and straight. Pull your navel in toward your spine. Bend your elbows a little more than 90 degrees and position them directly under your shoulders so that your upper arms are roughly perpendicular to the floor and close to your sides.

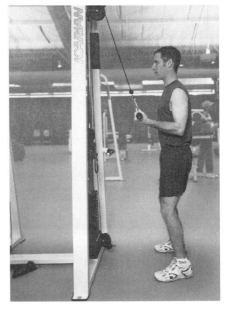

**Action:**
Keeping your upper arms stationary, pull the bar down toward your thighs until your elbows are almost straight. Return to the starting position in a slow, controlled manner.

**Variation:**
- ■ This exercise may also be done with one arm at a time, using a small handle.

**Tip:**
- ■ Do not allow any upper arm or torso movement.

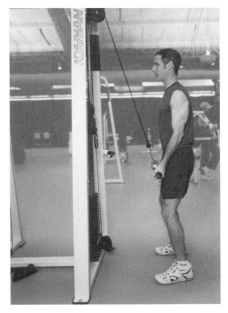

# CABLE TRICEPS OVERHEAD PRESS-OUT

**Muscle Group(s) Targeted:**
Back of the upper arm (triceps)

**Starting Position:**
Attach a bar or rope handle to the end of the cable in the high pulley position. Stand with your back to the cable unit, 1 to 2 feet away from the machine in a staggered stance. Bend forward slightly from your hips. Place your hands on top of the bar about shoulder width apart or grip the rope handles with your palms facing each other. Keep your head in line with your spine, your shoulder blades drawn together and down, a natural arch in your lower back, and your wrists firm and straight. Pull your navel in toward your spine. Bend your elbows 90 degrees or a little more and position them in front of and slightly higher than your shoulders.

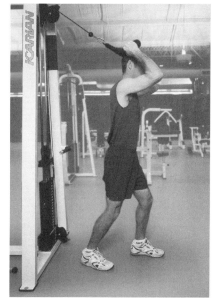

**Action:**
Keeping your upper arms still, press your arms forward until your elbows are straight. Return to the starting position in a slow, controlled manner.

**Variation:**
- Perform with one arm at a time, using the small, one-hand handle.

**Tips:**
- Keep your elbows no wider than shoulder width.
- Do not allow your torso, shoulders, upper arms, or wrists to move. All movement should occur at your elbows.

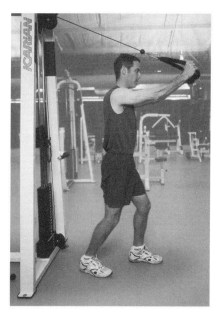

# 12. FOREARMS

## DUMBBELL OR BARBELL FOREARM (REVERSE) CURL

**Muscle Group(s) Targeted:**
Forearm and front of upper arm (brachioradialis and biceps)

**Starting Position:**
Stand with your feet approximately shoulder width apart and your knees slightly bent. Hold the dumbbells down at your sides with your palms facing behind you and your elbows slightly bent, or hold the barbell just in front of your thighs with the hands shoulder width apart and palms facing your thighs. Keep your focus forward, your shoulder blades drawn together and down, a natural arch in your lower back, and your wrists firm and straight. Pull your navel in toward your spine, and do not lock your elbows.

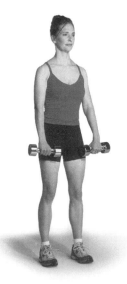

**Action:**
Bend your elbows, bringing the backs of your hands up toward your shoulders while keeping your elbows down at your sides, directly under your shoulders. Return to the starting position in a slow, controlled manner.

**Variations:**
■ You may do a dumbbell forearm curl while seated on a bench or stool.
■ With the dumbbell curl, you may do one arm at a time, alternating arms with each repetition or performing all repetitions with one arm first and then with the other arm.

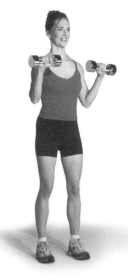

**Tips:**
■ Do not allow any shoulder movement. Keep your upper arms stationary.
■ Keep your trunk stationary. Do not allow any back and forth motion.

# TUBING FOREARM (REVERSE) CURL

**Muscle Group(s) Targeted:**

Forearm and front of upper arm (brachioradialis and biceps)

**Starting Position:**

Stand with your feet slightly apart, your knees slightly bent, and the center of the tubing under the arch of each foot. Place your arms down at your sides about shoulder width apart, your palms facing back with the elbows slightly bent. Hold one handle in each hand.

**Action:**

Bend your elbows, bringing the backs of your hands up toward your shoulders while keeping your elbows down at your sides, directly under your shoulders. Keep your focus forward, your shoulder blades drawn together and down, a natural arch in your lower back, and your wrists firm and straight. Pull your navel in toward your spine, and do not lock your elbows or knees. At the top of the motion, your palms should be facing forward. Return to the starting position in a slow, controlled manner.

**Variations:**

- Do one arm at a time, alternating arms with each repetition or performing all repetitions with one arm first and then with the other arm.
- Stand with one foot in front of the other with the center of the tubing under the arch of the front foot (less challenging).
- Stand off-center on the tubing and perform the exercise with the side that has the longer tubing length and then switch sides (less challenging).
- For increased resistance, place both handles in one hand and do each arm separately (more challenging).

**Tips:**

- Keep your upper arms stationary and next to the sides of your body without excessively pressing against your body.
- Do not allow any shoulder movement during the exercise.

### *Cooldown and Stretching*

Again, remember when you strength-train, you are really working those muscles hard, and it's extremely important that you take the best possible care of them by following every strength-training session with a cooldown and stretches. Here are a few new stretches that you might use following your non-foundation strength-training workout.

## CHEST AND UPPER BACK MUSCLES

### *Chest Stretch*

Stand or sit and clasp both hands behind your head with the elbows pointing out to the sides. Slowly pull your elbows back while expanding and lifting your chest outward and upward. Avoid arching the lower back excessively. Hold 20 seconds.

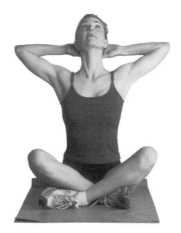

*Upper Back Stretch*

Stand with your feet shoulder width apart, knees slightly bent, your arms out in front of you, and your fingers interlocked, palms facing you. (This stretch may also be done seated or lying.) Slowly bring your hips and shoulders forward, press the center of your spine backward, and bend the knees so that your spine forms a C curve, with the front of your body concave and the back convex. Lower your head, keeping it in line with the spine. Press forward with your arms and pull back with your upper back until you feel a stretch across the upper back. Hold 20 seconds.

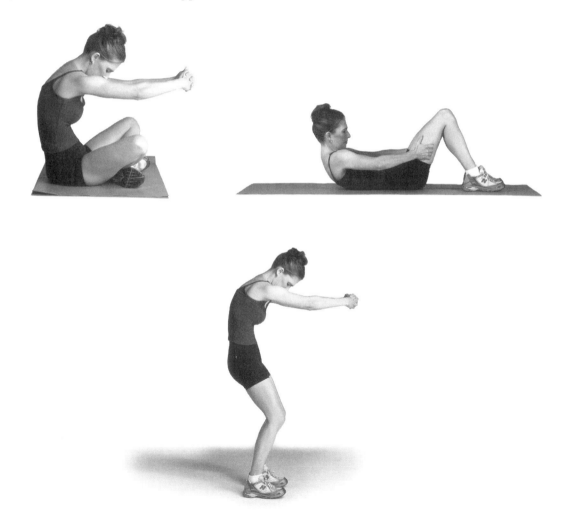

## SHOULDER MUSCLES

### *Shoulder Stretch*

Sit or lie and bring one arm across your body with the elbow straight and the arm parallel to the floor. Place the other hand just above the elbow on the upper arm and pull the arm in toward your chest. Hold 20 seconds and repeat on the other side.

Tip: Keep your shoulders down.

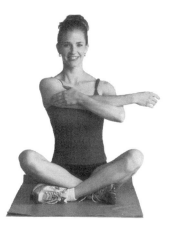

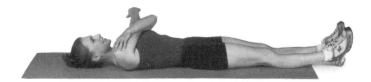

## SIDE AND NECK STRETCHES

*Sides-of-Torso Stretch*

Sit or stand erect and reach one arm high overhead. Slowly lean to one side and reach up and over with the arm of the side you are stretching. Your other arm may reach as well, or you may place it on your hip or thigh to stabilize yourself. Do not collapse the opposite side. Think of reaching upward as much as sideways. Hold 20 seconds and then stretch the opposite side.

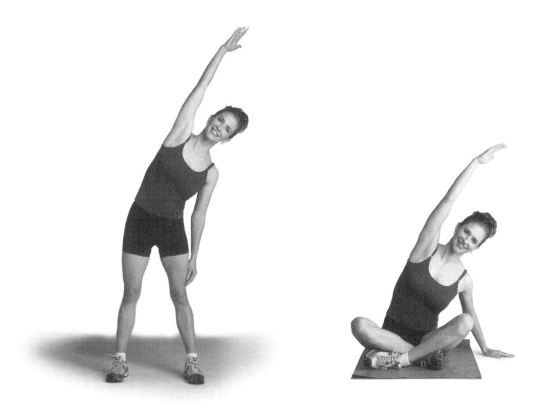

*Neck Sidebend and Stretch*

Start with your head in line with your spine and your focus forward. Turn your head a quarter turn to the left and, from that position, drop your chin toward your chest. Keep your other shoulder down. Hold 20 seconds and then stretch the opposite side.

Sitting comfortably or standing, look straight ahead and slowly lower one ear toward the shoulder. Do not pull on the head. If you need more stretch, lower the shoulder down on the opposite side. Hold 20 seconds and then stretch the opposite side.

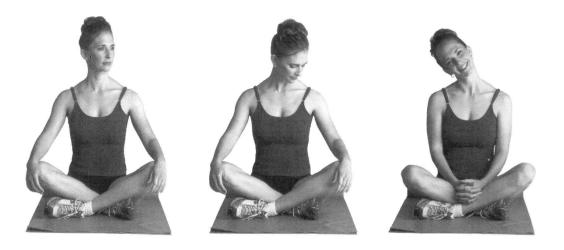

## STRETCHES FOR THE ARM MUSCLES

### *Triceps Stretch*

Bring one arm straight over your head until the upper arm is right next to your head. Bend your arm, dropping your hand behind your head and grasp that elbow with the opposite hand. Gently press the elbow back and toward the midline of the body until you feel a gentle stretch in the back of the upper arm. Hold 20 seconds and repeat on the other side.

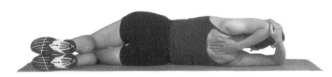

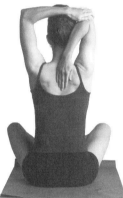

### *Biceps Stretch*

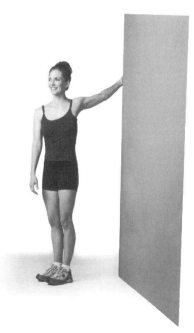

Sit or stand 2 to 3 feet away from a wall with your back to the wall. Rotate your upper body so that you can place your hand on the wall slightly above shoulder level with the fingers pointing sideways, away from you. Keeping the hand in place, gradually turn your upper body back toward the front until a stretch is felt along front of the upper arm. Hold 20 seconds and repeat on the other side.

*Top of the Forearm*

Stand or sit and lift one arm straight out in front of you with the palm facing down. Bend your wrist so that your fingers point toward the floor and your palm is facing you. Use your other hand to gently pull your hand toward you until you feel a mild stretch along the top of your forearm. Hold 20 seconds and repeat on the other side.

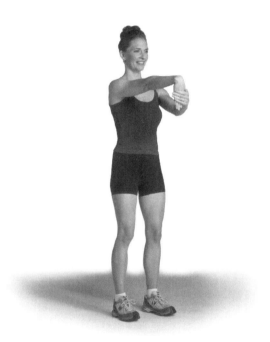

*Underside of the Forearm*

Stand or sit and lift one arm straight out in front of you with the palm facing up. Bend your wrist so that your fingers point toward the floor and your palm faces away from you. Use your other hand to gently pull your hand toward you until you feel a mild stretch along the top of your forearm. Hold 20 seconds and repeat on the other side.

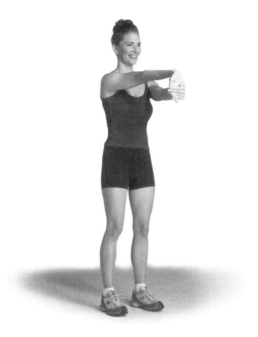

### The Next Step

Now I know you have followed the RealAge workout rules perfectly, and are walking 30 minutes every day come heck, earthquake, or high water. By now, too, you have added the foundation-strengthening exercises and are doing those every other day, plus the non-foundation exercises in this chapter and are doing these every other day as well. And by now you are wondering if you can finally start sweating with the stamina exercises. The answer is—not until you can check the following box:

> ❏ Yes, I did it! I have done the walking every day for 90 consecutive days, the foundation-strengthening exercises every other day for 60 days, and the non-foundation muscle strengtheners every other day for 30 days.

If you can check that box, great! By now, you are at least 60 percent of the way toward the age reduction you will get from the complete program. In other words, women will get about 5.7 years younger by doing just the walking and the weights, men about 5.4 years younger. Celebrate your accomplishment! Then, it's time to self-evaluate so that you can chart the progress you have made so far.

## Self-Evaluation at the End of Phase 3

It's been 3 months since your first assessment. Repeat it now (pages 24–25). For your retest, either you can change the weight you use for your 8 to 12 repetitions, or you can see how many repetitions you can perform with the original 8- to 12-repetition weight. If you choose to go to a new weight, you can use the following formula to estimate your percentage gain in strength:

$$\frac{(\text{weight 2} - \text{weight 1}) \times 100}{\text{weight 1}} = \underline{\quad} \%$$

weight 1 = weight used for first assessment
weight 2 = weight used for second assessment

If your strength has started to increase, you're ready for stamina. And that's great news. Chances are good you're going to get hooked on a fun and challenging new program of running, swimming, bicycling, or some other sport that will make you feel—and actually be—younger. You've done great work so far, and now it's time to enjoy all three types of exercise for maximum health and vitality. Go for it.

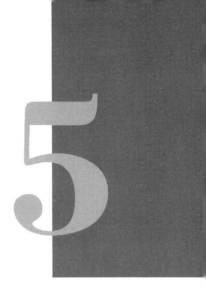

# Phase 4 (Days 91 Onward): Stamina

Once your schedule includes walking for at least 30 minutes every day for 90 days and strength-training activities every other day for at least 60 days, you are ready to move on to stamina activities. Actually, you're more than ready. The strength and general physical activities you have made part of your life have greatly reduced your risk of injury. That means that doing vigorous exercise will likely be fun.

Stamina activities—also called aerobic—are the activities we usually think of as exercise, such as jogging, stair climbing, biking, and swimming. Stamina activities train your heart, make your arteries more flexible and bolster the immune system. While the prospect of starting a stamina routine may feel daunting, it shouldn't be. Chances are you're going to end up loving this part of your RealAge Workout. Before you get started, however, I'd like you to do two things. First, I'd like you to pay a visit to your doctor. Explain to him or her that you're about to increase your activity from moderate to vigorous, and show him or her the following tests.

## An Evaluation of Your Fitness Capacity

Fitness capacity measures your body's reaction to vigorous exercise. If you evaluate your fitness capacity now, you can track your progress over the coming months as you incorporate stamina into your exercise routine. I guarantee that the changes you witness will be remarkable. Once you get the green light from your doctor, take the following three tests and record the results on your progress report sheet (pages 24–25). You will need a method of measuring your heart rate, such as a device that is built into the handles of many exercise machines, or the heart rate monitor watch and strap discussed on page 8.

These tests have resulted from studies done at the Cooper Clinic, The National Lipid Clinic Trial headquartered at Johns Hopkins, the Cleveland Clinic (my own clinic), and several other sites. Each of these tests can predict your risk of dying and disability in the next ten years from numerous causes (not just heart disease or arterial aging). However, you should use the result from only one table—the table that makes you the youngest. The results are not to be added together. By doing the tests, you will ascertain the following:

1. *Your ability to achieve 80 to 90 percent of the age-adjusted maximum heart rate with exercise for 3 minutes (see Table 5.1).* Your age adjusted maximum heart rate is 220 minus your calendar age. When you are performing the maximal exercise you are capable of, does your heart rate reach 80 to 90 percent of the maximum heart rate desirable for your age group?

2. *Your maximum exercise capacity in METs (see Table 5.2).* How strenuous an activity can you perform? That is, what is your exercise capacity in terms of METs? A MET is a measure of metabolic energy expended per minute—the more METs you can do, the greater your exercise capacity. An increase in exercise capacity relates to a greater energy production capability per minute because your mitochondrial energy plants (in your cells) and arteries have increased their capabilities. (We convert that number of METs to kilocalories per hour and per minute, because kilocalories is the unit listed on many/most exercise machines such as treadmills, bicycles, elliptical trainers, stair steppers, and rowing machines.)

## Table 5.1

### The RealAge Effect of Achieving 80 to 90 Percent of Age-Adjusted Maximum Heart Rate* with Exercise for 3 Minutes

For Men:
Ability to Achieve 80 to 90% of Age-Adjusted Maximum
Heart Rate with Exercise for 3 Minutes

| CALENDAR AGE | LESS THAN 80% | 80–89.9% | 90% or HIGHER |
|---|---|---|---|
| | | REALAGE | |
| 35 | 36.1 | 34 | 31.4 |
| 55 | 57.7 | 52.9 | 49.6 |
| 70 | 72.9 | 67 | 63.7 |

For Women:
Ability to Achieve 80 to 90% of Age-Adjusted Maximum Heart
Rate with Exercise for 3 Minutes

| CALENDAR AGE | LESS THAN 80% | 80–89.9% | 90% or HIGHER |
|---|---|---|---|
| | | REALAGE | |
| 35 | 36.7 | 34.0 | 31.4 |
| 55 | 57.7 | 52.4 | 49 |
| 70 | 73.1 | 66.2 | 63.2 |

* Your age-adjusted maximum heart rate is 220 minus your calendar age.

3. *Your heart rate recovery 2 minutes after maximal exercise (see Table 5.3. This recovery test may not be pertinent for those over 60.).* Right at the end of the most strenuous workout you do, note your heart rate and the rate of kilocalories you are burning per hour at peak. Then stop all exercise (this one time, and one time only, do not cool down) and check your heart rate 2 minutes later. Then do your normal cooldown and your usual stretches.

## Table 5.2

## The RealAge Effect of Your Maximum Exercise Capacity in METs

### For Men:
#### Maximum Exercise Capacity in METs

| LESS THAN 4.5 | 4.5– 7.6 | 7.7– 8.9 | 8.9– 10.9 | 11.0 or MORE |
|---|---|---|---|---|

#### Or Maximum Exercise Capacity in Kcals per Hour

| LESS THAN 400 | 400– 550 | 551– 650 | 651– 750 | 751 or MORE |
|---|---|---|---|---|

| CALENDAR AGE | REALAGE | | | |
|---|---|---|---|---|
| 35 | 36.1 | 35 | 34 | 32.8 | 31.4 |
| 55 | 57.7 | 55 | 52.9 | 51.3 | 49.6 |
| 70 | 72.9 | 70 | 67 | 65.3 | 63.7 |

### For Women:
#### Maximum Exercise Capacity in METs

| LESS THAN 4.4 | 4.4– 7.3 | 7.4– 8.5 | 8.6– 9.9 | 10.0 or MORE |
|---|---|---|---|---|

#### Or Maximum Exercise Capacity in Kcals per Hour

| LESS THAN 400 | 400– 550 | 551– 650 | 651– 750 | 751 or MORE |
|---|---|---|---|---|

| CALENDAR AGE | REALAGE | | | |
|---|---|---|---|---|
| 35 | 36.7 | 35 | 34.0 | 33.7 | 31.4 |
| 55 | 57.7 | 55 | 52.4 | 50.7 | 49 |
| 70 | 73.1 | 70 | 66.2 | 64.7 | 63.2 |

## Table 5.3
## The RealAge Effect of Heart Rate Recovery 2 Minutes After Maximum Exercise

For Men:
Heart Rate Recovery (Decrease in Beats Per Minute)
2 Minutes After Maximum Exercise

| | LESS THAN 22 | 22–52 | 53–58 | 59–65 | 66 or MORE |
|---|---|---|---|---|---|
| CALENDAR AGE | | | REALAGE | | |
| 35 | 36.1 | 35 | 34 | 32.8 | 31.4 |
| 55 | 57.7 | 55 | 52.9 | 51.3 | 49.6 |
| 70 | 72.9 | 70 | 67 | 65.3 | 63.7 |

For Women:
Heart Rate Recovery (Decrease in Beats Per Minute)
2 Minutes After Maximum Exercise

| | LESS THAN 22 | 22–52 | 53–58 | 59–65 | 66 or MORE |
|---|---|---|---|---|---|
| CALENDAR AGE | | | REALAGE | | |
| 35 | 36.7 | 35 | 34.0 | 33.7 | 31.4 |
| 55 | 57.7 | 55 | 52.4 | 50.7 | 49 |
| 70 | 73.1 | 70 | 66.2 | 64.7 | 63.2 |

If you achieved at least 90 percent of the maximum heart rate desirable for your age group, 751 kcal per hour peak maximum exercise, or your heart rate declined by 66 or more beats in the 2 minutes after you stopped, your RealAge is at least 5 years younger than your calendar age. If you are not there yet and want to make your RealAge younger, simply follow the RealAge Workout plan—you will get there.

## Warm-Up for Stamina Exercises

We've talked about warming up several times in this book, but it is important enough to touch on it again. Remember, the warm-up prepares your body physically and psychologically for your upcoming workout. Warming up is always important, but when you're doing intense stamina activity, a warm-up is especially important. That's because muscles heated by a warm-up become more flexible. This increased flexibility makes them more mechanically efficient during vigorous activity. It also lessens the chance of an injury. An elastic muscle can both stretch and absorb shock better than a stiff muscle.

Here are two great pre-stamina warm-ups:

1. Perform a moderate version of the exercise you're about to begin. For example, slow biking warms you up for intense biking, a slow jog prepares you for a faster jog, etc. If you are going to play basketball, work on the skills you're about to use: Dribble, pass the ball a few times, take some shots, run the court, jump in place, and if your aim is to be the next Michael Jordan, practice a few 360-degree dunks.

Follow with some range-of-motion activities, moving the joints you will be using in all directions they can safely move.

2. Perform a whole-body warm-up of a more creative nature:

■ Simultaneously swing each arm back and forth in opposite directions, and bend your knees during each swing through.

■ Gradually begin to circle your arms all the way around while continuing to move them in opposite directions. (That 360-degree dunk is probably beginning to feel easy.)

■ Next, swing your arms together from side to side in front of your body, leaning your torso in the direction of each swing and lunging slightly in that direction as well.

■ Once you have completed a few of these motions, begin traveling to one side in a "step-together-step" pattern as you swing the arms around in a full circle.

■ Reverse directions and repeat.

■ Follow this with a set of leg swings. Holding on to a wall or bar, balance on one leg. Keeping your spine erect and stable, swing your free leg forward and back (your knee can be slightly bent), moving only at the hip joint.

■ Next, swing your leg across your body and then out to the side.

■ Switch legs. You may decide how many of each swing to perform, but the entire sequence should last 5 minutes.

## The Workout

In this ultimate phase of the RealAge Workout, all you have to do is raise your heart rate to over 80 percent of your age-adjusted maximum (using a heart rate monitor for accuracy; your age-adjusted maximum is 220 minus your age). If this exercise makes you sweat in a cool room, you can also assume that your heart is beating at that rate. You should do this for 21 consecutive minutes 3 times a week.

An activity that causes you to sweat 21 minutes at a time has a double benefit: It not only counts toward the 63 minutes of stamina exercise required per week for optimum Age Reduction but also burns extra calories toward your goal of expending 3,500 kilocalories per week. Because of this double benefit, stamina exercises can make your RealAge as much as or even more than 7.4 years younger. Choose machines such as an elliptical trainer or an exercise bike that do not involve as much up-and-down pounding as running and you'll increase your odds that osteoarthritis will not keep you from continuing your age-reduction plan.

By definition, a stamina-building activity must meet the following criteria:

1. It must involve movement utilizing large muscle groups.
2. It must be continuous.
3. It must elevate your heart rate to more than 80 percent of age-adjusted maximum (220 minus your calendar age).

If you can, measure your heart rate every time you exercise for the first couple of months. You will eventually come to notice how your body feels at a given heart rate, and then you can switch to the RealAge Workout scale below, where you rely on your own perceptions to gauge your intensity. This method allows you to focus on the way you feel, while at the same time giving you a concrete sense of what that means in terms of your heart rate. Once you have completely switched over to the perceived exertion model, check your heart rate periodically to verify the accuracy of your perceptions.

### The RealAge Workout Scale

To help you gauge your level of intensity, I have developed a scale from 1 to 10. (You need to reach at least 6, and preferably 7, to be at the heart rate that gives you the most benefits from stamina activities.)

1. *Effortless.* How you might feel when reclining to watch television. There is no elevation in your breathing.
2. *Very light effort.* How you might feel brushing your teeth, shaving, or putting on makeup. There is no noticeable elevation in your breathing.
3. *Light effort.* You might experience this level while walking around the house. There is a slight elevation in your breathing, but you are probably not aware of it.
4. *Light to moderate effort.* When you go for a leisurely stroll, you may reach this level. Your breathing is noticeably elevated but still relatively slow and comfortable.
5. *Moderate effort.* You are on a brisk walk. You can still easily carry on a conversation, but you are aware that you are working. Your breathing rate and depth are increased.
6. *Moderately heavy effort.* You walk as quickly as possible. You know you are breathing harder, but at the same time you know you can continue at this pace for a while. You begin to perspire lightly.
7. *Heavy effort.* You are breathing faster and deeper, and you are perspiring. You could still carry on a conversation, but you'd rather not. This is likely where you will spend much of your stamina-exercising time.
8. *Very heavy effort.* You are exercising so vigorously that you are not sure you can keep up this pace for the next 15 minutes. You can converse only in short phrases. You have a feeling of discomfort (but not necessarily of a negative sort).

9. *Extreme effort.* You are exercising at your peak, and must concentrate to keep up this intensity. You feel you cannot do it for long. Many professional athletes train in this range, but it is unnecessary for the rest of us.

10. *Maximum effort.* Most exercisers never reach this level, and it is not advisable to try to do so.

If you take beta-blockers, calcium channel blockers, nitrates, or thyroid medications (this is only a partial list), you may have an atypical heart rate both while resting and during exercise. In this case, you should measure your intensity based on the RealAge Workout scale rather than on the heart-rate-based scale. Monitor your heart rate to become familiar with your average rate at any given exertion level or fitness level.

Maximum fitness is different from maximum health benefit. Nevertheless, when you are gaining a maximum health effect from physical activity, you will usually attain a high fitness level based on the following scale:

■ *Low fitness level* (sedentary or has clinical conditions)—Start with an intensity of 55–65 percent (4 to 5 on the RealAge scale) of your maximum heart rate (220 minus your age). Then move up when you feel you can, but not faster than a 10 percent increase in any week or any session no matter how good you feel.

■ *Moderate fitness level* (active)—65–80 percent of your maximum HR (6 on the RealAge scale). And then move another notch higher.

■ *High fitness level* (exercises regularly)—80–90 percent of your maximum HR (7 to 8 or higher on the RealAge scale).

Once you have reached your cardiorespiratory fitness goal, you may enter what many call the maintenance phase of your program. Some fitness professionals balk at this term, claiming that if you are not progressing you are really moving backward. This is not so. The body's natural course is to become less and less fit over time. After age 35, the average person will experience a 5 percent decline each decade in muscle mass, cardiorespiratory function, IQ—every function we can measure.

By maintaining your fitness level when you are doing all three activities for maximum RealAge benefit, you are in a very real sense progressing. The distance between where you are now physically and where you would be without exercise continues to grow.

### *Your Stamina Training Options*

There are two approaches my patients use to choose their stamina activity once they have committed to this fourth phase of the RealAge Workout. One is to rediscover the joy of a sport they used to love but haven't done for a while whether because of family responsibilities, a job, or because they've simply gotten out of shape, or to engage in an activity they have never done before, such as cardio kick-boxing or in-line skating. I encourage this approach as much as possible—there are enough great choices that everyone can find (or rediscover) a stamina activity they genuinely love. The second approach you may have to use from time to time—and that some people use all the time—is to consider stamina activity a job. They state: "There are plenty of days I'd rather not go to work, yet I still go because that is my job." Some days even enjoyable activities will fall into this category. No matter what approach you take—and it may well be a combination of the two—you have plenty of great options.

So what stamina activities should *you* participate in? Deciding may take some time. The more muscles you can involve in your stamina-building activities, the fitter you will be. You may have to try a few in order to find out which you really love. And don't think you can know what you like best after trying something for only 2 minutes. You should test-drive each piece of equipment for no less than the time you plan on using it—at least 21 minutes and at least 3 times, which means you'll probably need to go to the gym or hit the playing field more than once.

Other issues to consider when choosing are:

### WHAT ARE YOUR FITNESS GOALS?

If you want to participate in a backpacking tour through Europe, you probably should not make swimming your primary stamina-building activity.

### DO YOU LIKE TO BE ALONE OR ARE YOU A TEAM PLAYER?

Some activities may isolate you more than others, and you should choose according to your preference. You may choose a combination of solitary and group activities. As you probably train differently in a secluded setting than you do in a more social one, a combination of both may be beneficial.

## IS THERE A REASON YOU SHOULD NOT PARTICIPATE IN CERTAIN ACTIVITIES?

If running aggravates the arthritis in your knees, you may need to choose a seated activity, such as stationary biking, rowing, or recumbent stepping. Swimming may also be a good choice.

## DO YOU LIKE TO BE OUTDOORS OR INSIDE?

Some people love to be out in the sunshine and fresh air; others like to stay inside to avoid the elements. Let's look at some of the options available to you, depending on your preferences.

### *Outdoor Activities*

#### RUNNING

- Calorie-burning potential (by which we mean keeping your heart rate over 80 percent of your age-adjusted maximum for 21 minutes 3 times a week): high
- Injury rate: moderately low to high, depending on intensity, mileage, and running surface
- Main advantages: reasonably inexpensive; convenient; requires shorter duration
- Cautions/disadvantages: requires proper shoes; high degree of stress on weight-bearing joints and ligaments; need to avoid cement surfaces

Runners love their sport. If you ask them why they run, 90 percent will let their tongues run away on a marathon talking spree as they enumerate the countless physical, spiritual, and philosophical virtues of running. However, running can be unwise and uncomfortable for many people with musculoskeletal conditions. Protect your joints from excess strain with great running shoes (which you replace as soon as they have given you 350 miles of service or after 6 months, whichever comes first) and jog on surfaces such as rubberized asphalt, grass, and dirt trails that absorb shock. Also, limit your mileage. Running over 35 miles per week greatly increases the risk of injury. If you are a beginner, start with a walk/jog program. Once you can jog continuously for a few minutes at a time, gradually increase your running time and then gradually increase your speed.

## CYCLING

- Calorie-burning potential: low to high
- Injury rate: low, with the exception of accidents
- Main advantages: little stress on weight-bearing joints; develops proprioception
- Cautions/disadvantages: requires a good, reliable bike with multiple gears (aim for at least 10); must have proper seat height; helmet required; avoid traffic and slippery or unstable terrain

Outdoor cycling is easy to do with a friend or group of friends, and once people get out on their bikes, they tend to exercise for a longer period of time than those who choose other activities. Be careful of going too fast—even Lance Armstrong takes a spill now and then. A good bike can also be expensive. Before buying, test out rentals for several weeks and seek the advice of an experienced bike shop owner. And wear a helmet!

## SWIMMING

- Calorie-burning potential: usually moderate (to gain the same stamina benefit, I've been told swimmers need to do 80 percent of maximum minus 10 beats per minute, but I can find no substantiating data)
- Injury rate: low
- Main advantages: minimal stress on joints; uses upper and lower body muscles
- Cautions/disadvantages: requires a high level of motor skill before you can get a good stamina-building workout (unless you take a water aerobics class); often not convenient; seasonal (if outdoors); can aggravate a shoulder condition

Expect to take time learning correct form. Swimming requires a high level of technique and, therefore, practice. Work with a swimming coach at least once. If you are a beginner, start with an interval-training workout—that is, swim a couple of pool lengths and then walk for a while. Over time, your endurance will build and your stroke will become more efficient, enabling you to swim continuously for an entire workout at a heart rate that provides RealAge stamina benefits.

## ROWING

- Calorie-burning potential: high
- Injury rate: low
- Main advantages: easy on weight-bearing joints; develops arms, back, and thigh endurance and strength (depending on resistance)
- Cautions/disadvantages: requires some practice; may aggravate shoulder or elbow conditions; often not convenient to do outdoors; can be seasonal (but I love the Concept II indoor rowing machine, which fits conveniently into a small space and provides great stamina workouts all year); may be expensive

What could be nicer than an excellent workout gliding across water on a beautiful day? Sure, working out on a StairMaster on the top deck of your yacht meets this description, but we're talking rowing here. To reap stamina-building rewards, your rowing must be more rigorous than the basic "row, row, row . . . gently down the stream." Done properly, rowing, which develops the upper body without overburdening the weight-bearing joints, is an ideal cross-training exercise (see cross-training, page 171).

## SKATING/ROLLERBLADING

- Calorie-burning potential: moderate to high
- Injury rate: low, with the exception of accidents. About one in twenty-five skaters ends up in the emergency room each year due to a skating injury, most commonly a fractured wrist or arm.
- Main advantages: less stress on joints than running
- Cautions/disadvantages: requires a moderately high level of balance and

motor skills; need to wear a helmet, wrist guards, and elbow and knee pads; avoid traffic

Participants hail skating as an all-season, socially rewarding, inexpensive, challenging, and effective activity as well as a good source of transportation. Thirty minutes of skating at a moderate pace burns roughly 285 calories and generates an average heart rate of 148 beats per minute. Skating provides a better aerobic workout than cycling because you cannot coast as much while skating. (Running is better still because you cannot coast at all.)

## CROSS-COUNTRY SKIING

■ Calorie-burning potential: high
■ Injury rate: low
■ Main advantages: little stress on joints; inexpensive compared to downhill skiing
■ Cautions/disadvantages: requires high level of motor skill and coordination; seasonal; may not be convenient

Cross-country skiing, an exhilarating sport—to say the least, if you believe the enthusiasts who burst with happiness as they describe their run to you—provides lots of opportunities for social interaction, unless, of course, you decide to ski alone. It yields superior cardiorespiratory benefits without the considerable risk of injury associated with other high-intensity sports. This combination makes it one of the best exercises around.

As for the indoor version popularized by the NordicTrack, cross-country ski machines seem to inspire more sworn devotion and more intense disdain than any other class of equipment. Why the great divergence? Our theory is that some people (the devotees) quickly master the coordination, rhythm, and movement required for smooth and comfortable use of the machines, while others (the disdaining) do not.

## GAMES: BASKETBALL, SOCCER, LACROSSE, FIELD HOCKEY, BADMINTON, VOLLEYBALL, TENNIS, FOOTBALL, RACQUETBALL, SQUASH, ETC.

- ■ Calorie-burning potential: high
- ■ Injury rate: high, since most stress the knee with frequent twisting actions
- ■ Main advantages: so much fun that you hardly know you are doing physical activity; conditions almost all major muscle groups
- ■ Cautions/disadvantages: requires skill and partners/opponents of nearly equal skill level

### *Indoor Activities*

## TREADMILL WALKING *(at a fast pace, and at an incline— the higher the better)* OR RUNNING

- ■ Calorie-burning potential: moderate to high
- ■ Injury rate: low to moderate
- ■ Main advantages: requires shorter duration to hit the 80 percent heart rate goal because of the higher intensities; shock-absorbing surface; not seasonal
- ■ Cautions/disadvantages: can be expensive and takes up a lot of space; may be inconvenient if you must go to the gym to use one; requires good running (walking) shoes

Treadmills are the most popular stamina-building machines purchased for home use. Walking on a treadmill beats walking outdoors in one way: at any moment, you can incline your treadmill and enjoy uphill walking, dramatically increasing the intensity of your workout. Take advantage of this feature to have a challenging aerobic workout comparable to jogging with less stress to your joints. Jogging works well for short runs or interval training. Most decent treadmills feature shock-absorbing systems that make their surfaces easier on the joints than pavement or cement. Even so, you should limit your mileage to 35 miles per week.

## STATIONARY CYCLING

■ Calorie-burning potential: moderate to high

■ Injury rate: low

■ Main advantages: little stress on weight-bearing joints; safe; can usually adjust the resistance; not seasonal; little skill necessary

■ Cautions/disadvantages: May be boring; may be inconvenient if you must go to the gym; need proper seat position

Home stationary bikes are woefully underused because few riders learn to employ basic boredom-busting tactics (my favorite is watching comedy monologues I've missed—see other techniques on page 173). Many beginning cyclists attack the activity with too much gusto, burning out after 5 minutes, and conclude that cycling is "too hard," and many bike purchasers do not try out enough different models to determine the type they enjoy most (I like ones where both arm and leg movements are employed).

## JUMPING ROPE

■ Calorie-burning potential: high

■ Injury rate: moderately high

■ Main advantages: convenient; inexpensive; works arms and legs; not seasonal; can be done anywhere

■ Cautions/disadvantages: high stress impact on weight-bearing joints; hard to continue for long durations; requires fairly high level of motor skill and coordination

Jumping rope burns lots of calories quickly. It can be done just about anywhere, and is energizing and fun. The most portable piece of stamina-building equipment on the market, a jump rope is great for travel.

Before you begin jumping rope, learn a few different types of jumps so that you can alternate your routine. Avoid jumping if you are not yet moderately fit or if you suffer from a muscle or joint condition that could be worsened by the activity. Jumping rope can significantly accelerate your stamina-building progress. (I love jumping rope, but it does its best work as a secondary, rather than a primary, stamina-building exercise.)

## STAIR-CLIMBING

- ▓ Calorie-burning potential: moderate to high
- ▓ Injury rate: fairly low
- ▓ Main advantages: convenient (staircase, machines, or step board); fairly low impact on joints; does not require a high level of skill; not seasonal
- ▓ Cautions/disadvantages: do not support your weight on the guardrails; stop when you feel fatigued in order to avoid a fall or injury; use proper step height if using a step board

As the quotable Joan Welsh puts it, "A man's health can be judged by what he takes two at a time—pills or stairs." Stair-climbing can give you a great workout. But beware: As with any stamina-building activity, do not do so much of it that you injure yourself. Start with just 3 to 5 minutes and gradually "climb" from there.

## ELLIPTICAL MACHINES

- ▓ Calorie-burning potential: moderate to high
- ▓ Injury rate: low
- ▓ Main advantages: low stress impact on the joints; not seasonal; some models use both upper and lower body muscles
- ▓ Cautions/disadvantages: fairly expensive and space gobbling; may be inconvenient if you need to go to a gym

These machines combine the back-and-forth action of ski machines with the up-and-down action of stair climbers into a fluid semicircular motion. Some models feature inclining ramps for the legs but offer no resistance for the arms, while others provide arm handles but no incline feature. Choose the one that feels the best to you.

## REBOUNDING *(MINI-TRAMPOLINE)*

- ▓ Calorie-burning potential: moderate to high
- ▓ Injury rate: low to moderate (take some lessons first)

■ Main advantages: low stress on joints; inexpensive; can store easily; not seasonal; wide variety of movements possible

■ Cautions/disadvantages: use proper shoes (cross-trainers); need proper ventilation (breeze from a window or fan)

The mini-trampoline has reclaimed its maiden name, the rebounder, and divorced itself from exclusive home usage. Home rebounders can follow along with a rebounding video to learn all the up-to-date moves. Wherever you choose to park your trampoline, rebounding affords a great workout.

## AEROBIC DANCE

■ Calorie-burning potential: moderate to high

■ Injury rate: low to high, depending on the type and level of class (low or high impact)

■ Main advantage: group support and motivation; inexpensive; not seasonal; large amount of variety possible; can be low stress on the joints

■ Cautions/disadvantages: class schedule may be inconvenient; requires proper footwear (aerobic shoes); requires motor skills and coordination; target heart rate may be slightly higher; avoid hand weights

An aerobic dance class or video is only as good as the instructor. The relatively high level of concentration that an aerobics class requires is one of its most beneficial side effects. You can effectively operate a stair climber or stationary bike for a long period of time while your mind wanders and works its way through all of your problems, deadlines, and unfinished projects. On the other hand, an effective aerobic dance class will demand your attention, and will therefore give you a much-needed respite from the stresses of everyday life.

### Avoiding Injury

You are more likely to experience physical limitations and disabilities if you forgo physical activity than if you engage in it regularly. That said, exercise-related injury should be avoided at all costs. Injury frequently brings with it discouragement that leads to an abandoned exercise program. You don't want that. To minimize your risk of injury:

1. *Progress slowly and gradually.* Do not, even if you feel better than you ever have, increase your duration or intensity by more than 10 percent per week.
2. *Follow the 2-hour pain rule.* If you experience more pain than usual for more than 2 hours after exercise, you probably overdid it and should decrease the intensity and/or the amount of activity the next time you exercise.
3. *Learn your limits and honor them.* If you find yourself in the middle of a pain flare-up, don't hesitate to ease back. If you feel unusually tired or uncomfortable, rest.
4. *Avoid overtraining.* Overtraining occurs when your volume of training exceeds your body's ability to recover from that training. To avoid overtraining, you should vary the exercises you choose as well as the duration and intensity of training. Do not expend more than 6,500 kcals per week in physical activity.

If you exercise at a high level of intensity most days of the week, watch for symptoms of overtraining. They include loss in strength, fatigue, decreased appetite, illness, poor sleep patterns, muscle soreness, and decreased or increased resting heart rate and blood pressure. You may experience some of these symptoms occasionally as part of any exercise program—especially the fatigue and muscle soreness—but they should be short-lived. You could also be suffering from overtraining while not experiencing every symptom on the list. Listen to your body and give it the rest it needs. You cannot trade it in for a new one.

### Cross-Training

Cross-training is exactly what it sounds like: performing more than one stamina-building activity. Everyone should cross-train. You alternate the way you use your muscles and joints, decreasing your chances of sustaining overuse injuries. Cross-training also improves your cardiorespiratory fitness in ways that no single exercise can. It makes use of different muscles, which improves your overall conditioning. It makes a lot of sense for its health effect, and it is beneficial for its fitness effect.

Before embarking on a cross-training program, think about exercises that will complement one another—that is, use different muscles and body parts. If, for instance, you select a high-impact activity, such as running, as your primary stamina-building exercise, you could balance out your program with a low-impact activity (perhaps cycling, swimming, or rowing). Or if you choose rowing as your primary activity, you may want to select a secondary activity that utilizes more of the lower body, such as stair climbing. Develop a program that provides balance and decreases your risk of injury.

### Aerobic Interval Training

Another great way to add variety to your workout is with interval training. Interval training mixes short resting periods and/or short periods of low-intensity effort with bouts of high-intensity exercise in one training session. Most exercisers should incorporate interval training into their stamina-building programs. You do not need to follow a rigid interval program. Develop one that works for you. Adding breaks to a high-intensity workout or adding intense moments to a lower-intensity workout allows you to periodically recover mentally and physically. It also helps to relieve boredom. And interval training enables you to develop about the same level of aerobic proficiency that continuous, high-intensity training would provide.

### Use Weight to Your Advantage

If you are overweight, make the most of your excess pounds by choosing activities that require you to support your weight. Some terrific ones include walking, jogging, stair climbing, cross-country skiing, elliptical machine exercise, and rebounding (the mini-trampoline). If possible, make one or two of these activities your primary stamina exercises. You may supplement your program with swimming, biking, or rowing, but make these activities where you do not support your weight a supplement. Alternatively, if you are so overweight that fast walking, climbing stairs, aerobic dance classes, or other weight-bearing activities are uncomfortable, choose activities that take some of the weight off your legs. Try water exercise (even just walking in waist-to chest-deep water) or use a recumbent bike, which allows you to work out while sitting. You can gradually work up to weight-bearing activities.

*Fighting Boredom*

It helps to learn techniques to overcome boredom so that you can maintain your stamina routine over the long haul. If you climb onto the same stationary bike in the same room and pedal for the same number of RPMs at the same intensity for the same amount of time day after day, staring at a blank wall, boredom may eventually make you give up.

There are several ways to keep your workout from getting boring. You might mix it up by exercising with a friend, partner, or group. You might enter community events such as walkathons, triathlons (if you're in very good shape and want to push yourself), fun runs, and cycling races. You could watch TV, listen to the radio or a CD or iPod, or read (during lower-intensity workouts). You could even play games.

Play games? Sure—why not? Here are a few:

## A. "CHANGE THE RULES, BUT WORK THE SAME"

Select two variables that affect exercise intensity and manipulate them so that as one variable increases, the other decreases, and your work output remains the same.

Example: If you are riding a stationary bike for 21 minutes, you may start with a resistance level of 3.5 and perform 45 revolutions per minute, making your work output 150 watts. Every minute you might decrease the resistance by .1 and increase the RPMs so that your work output remains at 150 watts. By the end of the 21 minutes, you would be at a resistance of 1.6 and going at a pace of perhaps 80 RPMs, depending on the machine.

When using a treadmill, either increase the speed and decrease the incline or decrease the speed and increase the incline every couple of minutes. Even though your intensity remains quite steady, you have changed the variables and added variety, so the workout feels different.

## B. "JACK AND JILL WENT UP THE HILL"

The workload in this workout continues to increase until the last 2 to 5 minutes, during which the workload remains at its peak. You have to plan this one a bit, so you aren't at an impossibly high intensity only 5 minutes into the activity. If you plan on stair climbing for 21 minutes, you might decide to start on level 3. You know from past experience that you can handle level 8 for a few minutes, and that level 9 can last no more than 3 minutes. This means there are 6 level changes you can make in 17 to 18 minutes. (These are RealAge intensity levels, not levels on the machine.) The workout might go something like this:

| MINUTES SINCE START | LEVEL |
|---|---|
| 0–2 | 3 |
| 2–4 | 4 |
| 4–6 | 5 |
| 6–10 | 6 |
| 10–14 | 7 |
| 14–18 | 8 |
| 18–21 | 9 |
| 21–23 | cooldown |

This works in part because you are at the lowest effort needed when you have the most time left. As the intensity required increases, the time remaining decreases, giving you the mental power to finish.

### C. "I CAN DO ANYTHING FOR 30 SECONDS"

The high-intensity intervals are indeed high intensity, but only for 30 seconds each. The 30-second time limit makes a doable challenge, and the changes make it fun. You choose the length and intensity of your recovery intervals. Mine usually range from a minute to two at moderate to moderately high intensities.

### D. "THE TRIGGER SWITCH"

For this workout, pick a randomly occurring event that serves as a trigger to make you change your workout—either in intensity or the action of two variables that affect each other in terms of intensity. For example, the stair climber on the twelfth floor of my Chicago club faces Lake Michigan, Millennium Park, streets, and apartments. I pick an outside event to govern my workout.

For example, "Every time a red car goes by heading north, I will increase the intensity level by 1 until I reach level 9. Then I will reduce the level every red car until level 4, and then I will go back up again." Depending on traffic, I may go through 5 up-and-down cycles in 21 minutes or I may not get quite through a full cycle. I never know exactly what will happen, and I thrive on that uncertainty and surprise.

If it's a day when lots of sailboats are out on the lake, I may decide that every time a sailboat goes behind or appears from behind a certain apartment building I will change the way I am stepping. For example, I may rotate among baby steps, deep steps, and stepping with no hands touching the side rails. Choose your own triggers, depending on the surrounding environment, and choose the variables you will change when that trigger appears.

### A Word About the "Games"

You may be thinking, But you wrote to keep my heart rate at a 6–7 intensity for 21 minutes. Some games have my heart rate going all over the place! You're right. I have provided guidelines based on research that are effective and safe. But remember that they are *guidelines,* that variety is the spice of life (except in spouses), and that what is *most* important is that you move. If games increase your enjoyment of exercise (or help you tolerate it on bad days), use them. Don't take the RealAge Workout guidelines as rigid formulas (except for the 30-minute walking rule—that's non-negotiable). Make your exercise fun.

### Keeping Up Stamina Activity While Traveling

While travel inevitably alters your exercise routine, it need not stop it. Instead, it's another chance to introduce variety into your usual routine. Travel gives you the perfect opportunity to try something new or different—whether that may be an unexplored running path, a weight machine you've never tried, or a different type of cardio equipment (like Cynthia W. from Chapter 1 did with the elliptical trainer). Start looking at travel as a way to throw extra excitement and unpredictability into your workouts.

To ensure that your workouts actually happen, follow the Boy Scout motto and be prepared. Either look into the exercise opportunities where you will be staying ahead of time, or take what you'll need to do an "anytime, anyplace" workout.

Take advantage of resources. Begin by checking your hotel. Many have small but adequate gyms that provide the ultimate in convenience, and many have swimming pools. If you prefer an off-site health club, ask the hotel staff for a suggestion or log onto www.healthclubs.com. This site will give you the locations of nearby clubs as well as a list of their services and an estimated cost for a onetime visit. If you travel frequently and prefer this health club option, you can purchase a "club passport" that allows you to visit any participating IHRSA (International Health, Racquetball, and Sports Association) club at a discount rate. You may also want to purchase a membership at a large chain such as Bally or 24-Hour Fitness to be able to visit multiple locations at no charge.

Or bring along a DVD or VCR workout you can play on your laptop or TV in your hotel room, travel with a jump rope, or simply walk briskly around the hotel vicinity. Of course, you can also take advantage of the swimming pool if the hotel has one.

To enjoy the outdoors, ask about local hiking, running, or biking possibilities. The website www.trails.com contains an excellent listing of trails of all types. It also gives you the location, a description, the level of difficulty, the length of the trail, and a phone number to call if you want more information.

Finally, make it clear to your company, your travel companions, and the people you are meeting with that physical activity is a priority for you. Try to engage others in your activity. Set up a squash or tennis match. Go hiking. Staying active will make you more effective in your work and might influence others to be more active and healthy, too.

## The Cooldown

Never skip the cooldown. Think of it as an essential part of the stamina-building session. Stopping an intense activity too abruptly may increase your chances of experiencing heart arrhythmias. It also hinders the removal of lactic acid. Thus, not cooling down may make you feel very sore the next day.

Think of it this way: If you are driving a manual transmission automobile at 75 miles per hour in fifth gear, as you approach your final destination you can either (1) ease up on the gas and shift down, gear by gear, allowing the gears to slow your car before you press on the brakes and come to a gentle stop, or (2) you can step on your brakes while you are in fifth gear and let the brakes do all of the work.

Either way, you successfully stop your car, but in the first instance—the one in which you protect your car with a gradual cooldown before you come to a stop—you inflict a lot less wear and tear on your brakes. It's the same with exercise. Whereas the warm-up shifts your body into gear for vigorous physical activity, the cooldown and stretching shift your body gradually back down, allowing you to make a smooth re-entry into your everyday activities.

### Stretching

As you must know by now, I believe stretching after a workout should be mandatory. Stretching gives your body and mind time to relax and further cool down from the prior workout.

### Staying on Course

So there you have it—the four-part (warm-up, 21 minutes at 80 percent of peak age-adjusted heart rate, cooldown, stretching) stamina workout that constitutes the ultimate phase of your RealAge Workout. After 30 days, retake the fitness capacity test at the start of this chapter. Then take a moment to celebrate your progress. Most of all, have the peace of mind of knowing that—with your walking, your strength training, and your stamina building—you are engaged in the optimal workout to safeguard your health and your future. And there's every reason to continue for the rest of your life. After you've done 90 days of this phase, do another assessment. You will be over 8 years younger if you are a man and 9 years younger if a woman.

While you know so much more about fitness than you did when you started this book, you may still have questions. I'll try to answer them in the next chapter.

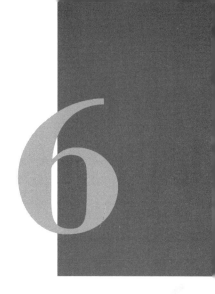

# Fitness FAQs

## Myth or Fact?

Truths, partial truths, and complete myths about physical activity and weight loss are everywhere. One statement you hear might contradict another. How are you to know what to believe?

To help you separate the truth from the myths, I have assembled the most frequently asked questions about exercise and answered them as best I—or my outside experts—can. Some of our answers are rock solid, substantiated by reams of scientific data. Others—and I'll identify which ones—are pure best *guesses*.

### I did all four phases of the RealAge Workout. When can I skip a day?

When it comes to walking, never (unless, of course, you're suffering from a broken leg or some other serious infirmity). Walk every day. With strength training, however, once you have hit maintenance (say, after 4 months of strengthening exercises), you only have to do strengthening once a week to maintain muscle mass (in fact, some recent data shows that strength training with a slow tempo—12 seconds per rep—once a week may make the strongest bones and muscles). But if you choose to do only one day a week for weight lifting, it is a much more challenging day than if you did it every other day. So I really believe every other day is the best and easiest way.

**I keep hearing that women have more body fat than men. If that's true, why should I even bother exercising?**

Until puberty, there are no significant differences in body composition or the percentage of body fat between girls and boys. During puberty, the higher levels of estrogen secretion in females increase fat deposits, especially in hips and thighs. This results in a higher percentage of body fat for women, on average, than for men. The average 30- to 49-year-old woman has 24–33 percent body fat, whereas the average man of the same age has 18–29 percent.

This should have nothing to do with whether or not you embark on a physical activity program. Exercise may not make you eager to be seen in a bikini (or it may), but it will increase your chance of having a higher quality of life with less disability—it reduces your chance of diabetes, heart attacks, strokes, memory loss, skin wrinkling, osteoarthritis, colon cancer, breast cancer, and many other conditions that may make your life less enjoyable. So physical activity almost certainly will increase your enjoyment of life. And you will realize that change in outlook quickly.

**Are men stronger than women?**

Yes, but not proportionately. The average man is 40–60 percent stronger in the upper body and 25–30 percent stronger in the lower body than the average woman. But men are generally larger to begin with and have more and larger muscle fibers than women. If we look at strength relative to fat-free mass, the differences largely disappear. Pound for pound of muscle, there's little or no difference between the strength of men and women. And a woman who lifts can be stronger, healthier, and younger than a man of the same chronological age who doesn't.

**Will I bulk up if I start lifting weights?**

Women, particularly, worry about bulking up, but this concern is unfounded. The strength-training routine in this book will probably make you "bulk down," as you become toned and your new muscles burn off excess fat. But even if you do bulk up a bit, those new muscles are a sign of increased vitality, and who wouldn't want that? Maybe it's time to stop viewing bulking up as something to avoid and start seeing it as a sign that you're getting younger.

This is not to say that you're going to look like Arnold any day soon. For those following a basic program of lifting 3 times a week for 10 to 20 minutes a session, the changes in visible muscle size will not be terribly dramatic. How much bulking up can you expect? The answer depends on genetics as well as the program, but here are a few general rules:

- Men, on average, appear to experience larger increases in muscle size than women, even if they perform similar training programs, but this apparent difference is deceptive. Men have more and larger muscle fibers (due somewhat to testosterone production in puberty) than women. When both genders undertake similar training programs, the percentage of enlargement of the muscles is about equal. It's just that a 10 percent increase in a big muscle appears much larger than a 10 percent increase in a small muscle.

- In general, lifting heavier weights causes more hypertrophy (larger muscles) than lifting lighter weights. Remember, you can avoid bulking up by using lighter weights and doing more repetitions, but doing so does not provide as much health benefit.

## How much weight will I lose by exercising?

Strength training is the lottery winner for weight loss. Consider that a pound of muscle uses 75 to 150 calories a day, and a pound of fat 1 to 3 calories a day. Since you normally lose 2 to 3 pounds of muscle every 10 years if you do not lift weights, you have to eat 150 to 450 calories less every day every 10 years just to keep the same weight. But weight lifting prevents that muscle loss and the weight gain that would otherwise accompany it. Your muscles use calories even when you are not doing weight lifting. This is one of many side benefits of building muscle.

Weight loss or weight gain is determined by the difference between the number of calories you consume and the number of calories you burn—that is, energy in versus energy out. Exercise is only one of many mechanisms that cause calories to be burned, and the number of calories you burn through exercise depends on multiple factors: (1) the amount of time you spend exercising, (2) the intensity at which you exercise, (3) the type of activity, and (4) your weight.

The longer you exercise, the more calories you burn. The more intensely you exercise, the more calories you burn. The more you weigh, the more calories you burn. The more muscle you utilize in the activity, the more calories you burn.

Though it is not possible to calculate exactly how much weight you will lose through exercise, we can give you a rough idea. A pound is equivalent to roughly 3,500 kilocalories. If you want to lose a pound of fat, you need to burn 3,500 calories more than you consume. (A calorie of food is the same unit as a kilocalorie of exercise—these are just the conventions for food and activity that have been adopted.) You could make losing a pound per week your goal. That would require that you maintain a 500-calorie-per-day deficit, so that in 7 days you would reach that 3,500-calorie deficit. But here's the thing to remember: You could accomplish this by reducing your calorie consumption by 200 calories a day and burning about 300 more calories per day through exercise.

But weight gain and weight loss are not as formulaic or cut-and-dried as they might seem. This type of calorie counting does not take into account changes in metabolism that may occur with exercise and dietary changes. It does not take into account the thermal effect of food and the calories required to digest it, and then to use or store it. Using the 3,500-calorie formula is a rough but acceptable guide.

**If I do leg lifts, will they burn the fat off my thighs? And will sit-ups take the fat off my abdomen?**

Unfortunately, spot reduction is a myth. You cannot determine which areas of the body lose fat in what proportions. Seen someone who has lost a lot of weight? They usually lose weight in the face first, and I know of few who do facial crunches. The best way to get rid of unwanted fat in any area is to do resistance exercises 3 times a week and engage in frequent stamina activity.

Also, avoid white foods (save cauliflower and fish and low- or non-fat dairy) as if white foods contain a malignant virus. Because white foods essentially are malignant viruses causing rapid increase in blood sugar and triglycerides, which make your arteries less able to dilate. And use 9-inch plates. Ironically, doing hundreds of leg lifts, lunges, or squats in the absence of a well-balanced exercise program is more likely to increase the definition in and size of your thigh by adding muscle. But what's wrong with more muscle? It looks and feels great!

## If I stop exercising, will my muscle turn to fat?

Muscle is muscle and fat is fat. They are two different types of tissue, and one will never turn directly into the other. If you stop physical activity, you are likely to lose some muscle and gain some fat, and since the fat accumulates to a degree where the muscle was, it makes it almost appear as if one turns into the other. To avoid this scenario, don't stop exercising. However, if you decrease the level of your activity, decrease your calorie consumption to compensate for the calories you are no longer burning. Too many athletes continue to eat like athletes once they have retired from competitive sports. That's why most football linemen gain 50 pounds or more the year after they retire. You see them two years later doing sports commentary, and you can hardly recognize them.

## Is it true that really fit people don't sweat as much as unfit people?

*(Weak data for this answer—so this is one of the best-guess answers.)* You have probably heard someone brag about how he or she doesn't sweat much during exercise. It's as if that person is insinuating that fit people don't sweat. Nothing could be more false. Sweating is the mechanism by which our bodies cool themselves. Without the ability to sweat, our body temperatures during stamina exercises could easily get hot enough to cause death.

Let's get scientific for a few moments. During exercise, our working muscles produce heat. Stamina exercise can increase heat production in the body by 15 to 20 times. The blood that flows through the muscles picks up the heat and carries it throughout the body, increasing your core temperature. When your brain senses the increased blood temperature, it directs the blood vessels by the skin to dilate, so that the blood can get close to the body's surface to be cooled off. You begin to sweat, and the evaporation of this sweat cools you off.

When you exercise regularly, your body gets more efficient at keeping itself cool. A fit person can keep his or her core temperature stable for longer than an unconditioned person, but as soon as the core temperature of a fit person begins to rise, he will start sweating much more quickly than his deconditioned counterpart. The unfit person may not begin to sweat until his body temperature has risen more than one degree. Fit people also distribute their sweat better, for a more optimum cooling efficiency, and their sweat is more dilute, meaning that they conserve more minerals.

### To see results from exercise, do I need to be in pain?

No. The important point to remember is that "pain is the messenger," and in this case the message is that you're overdoing it. Physical activity shouldn't be painful. True pain is your body's way of telling you to back off, slow down, and try a different regimen.

However, when you first start doing a physical activity, you may feel one kind of pain: a slow, burning ache in the muscles you haven't used in a while. This burning sensation you feel is actually good. It indicates you are reaching your anaerobic threshold, meaning you're at the limit of your endurance. The pain is believed to result from the buildup of lactic acid that occurs when your muscles are not getting enough oxygen (anaerobic means "in the absence of oxygen"). This burning is not an indication of an injury but a sign that you're doing what is optimal—"training at threshold."

Feeling sore after a workout does not mean that anything is necessarily wrong, especially if it occurs the next day. Unless you've actually sustained an injury, the pain will probably go away within a day or two, eventually producing lean muscle in place of flab.

### Am I too overweight to do physical activity?

Any trainer or doctor will tell you they often hear people say, "I'm too overweight to exercise." That's about as absurd as saying, "I'm too tired to rest," "I'm too hungry to eat," or "I'm too cold to put my sweater on."

Physical activity is exactly what you need if you are overweight. Excess body fat places the overweight person at an increased risk of developing the very conditions that cause aging—including high blood pressure, diabetes, arthritis, low back pain, sleep apnea, and their consequences, which cause aging of the arteries. Fat also ages your immune system, leading to an increase in autoimmune diseases, infections, and cancer. Weight loss reduces the stress on your knee joint by 7 times your loss in weight when going up stairs, and by 4 times when walking on a flat surface.

Weight loss also can have a positive impact on your social and emotional well-being. Reducing weight reduces accidents, injuries, and lower-back and joint pain, helping you enjoy life to the fullest.

## Can't I just diet?

Your body adjusts to diet alone by slowing its metabolic rate. So if you reduced your food intake by what is considered a pound's worth of calories—3,500 to be precise—and everything else stayed the same, you'd lose a pound for the first 3,500. By the tenth 3,500, however, you'd lose only seven-eighths of a pound, and progressively less. You need physical activity to maintain your metabolic rate in the face of reduced calorie intake.

If you weigh a lot, you start, in a sense, with an advantage. All of us burn about 20 percent more calories when standing than sitting. The more you weigh, the more calories you burn when you support that weight by standing.

Walking is the place to start. It's rare that you'll row from the parking lot to the office, bike around the mall, or swim from your kitchen to your bedroom. Outdoor transportation aside, you generally get around by supporting and moving your weight. And moving your body makes your RealAge younger.

## Will creatine as a supplement help my muscles become bigger faster?

Yes, but only a little of the size gain is due to real muscle—most is due to water accumulation. In some studies, creatine supplementation increases power, some report increases in speed, and some studies report no changes. In general, studies indicate that having some simple sugar immediately at the end of exercise and some protein seems to help muscles recover faster.

## So should I have a sports drink after my workout?

While you probably do not *need* a sports drink, you may benefit from one. If you think sports drinks are good-for-nothing, overpriced, artificially colored bottles of sugar water, you are partially right, but only partially—even fully priced and artificially colored sports drinks have some merit in the exercise world.

For exercise sessions lasting 30 minutes or less, plain water is perfect for rehydrating your body. For events lasting 60 minutes or more, sports drinks have a definite advantage over water. They rehydrate your body faster than water alone after long periods of exercise, helping you recover glycogen and muscle power sooner. They work faster because absorption of salt and sugar from the drink drags water across your intestine into your bloodstream. In addition, the minerals in sports drinks keep you from producing as much urine as drinking water alone would, so you do not lose as much fluid. Finally, both the flavor and the sodium in sports drinks keep you drinking longer than you might otherwise, so you are more likely to stay hydrated.

### To build larger muscles, should I eat more protein or take protein supplements?

Exercise does increase protein needs but usually not much. Proteins are necessary for the building and repairing of muscle, but most Americans ingest far more protein than they need—about 50 percent more than the needed 0.8 grams of protein per day per kilogram or 2 pounds of body weight (about 56 grams or 2 ounces of protein a day is what is needed).

To estimate the grams of protein you should consume in a day, multiply your weight in pounds by 0.4 to 0.8, depending on your physical status and activity level. If you are sedentary (which you'd better not be after reading this book) and healthy, multiply by 0.4. So on average, you need somewhere between 50 and 130 grams of protein a day. A 4-ounce serving of fish is a little more than 30 grams; 1 ounce of nuts is about 5 grams. If you are recovering from an illness or injury or are overstressed, multiply by 0.6. If you are pregnant, add 10 to 15 grams of protein per day to what you should normally have. If you are lactating, add 15 to 20 grams of protein per day to what you should normally have. If you are a moderate exerciser, multiply your weight in pounds by 0.6 to 0.7. If you are a strength and stamina fanatic, multiply by 0.75 to 0.9. Athletes who focus on building strength and muscle consume twice as much as the usual amount—1.6–1.7 grams of protein each day per kilogram of body weight to increase size of muscle and speed of recovery by 10 to 30 percent. This means that a 200-pound (90 kilogram) athlete should have about 150 grams (5 ounces) of protein per day. One small chicken breast contains 50 to 55 grams (about 2 ounces), so it doesn't take much food to get all your needs. Telling body builders that more protein than that does not help them is like telling a baby not to cry, but that's the scientific data.

### Someone told me that if I exercise too hard, I am no longer burning fat. Myth or fact?

Myth. This myth, however, has roots in science. When you exercise, the air you breathe out tells something about the type of fuel you are using. As exercise intensity increases, the typical body utilizes a higher percentage of carbohydrate-fueled, than fat-fueled, energy. Some incorrectly interpret this to mean as you increase exercise intensity, you are no longer burning fat, but only carbohydrates.

Wrong! The more you train, the more efficient your body becomes at using fat, so even at higher intensities you rely less on carbohydrates than when you were a couch potato. Since the total number of calories burned during higher-intensity exercise is larger than the number of calories burned during lower intensities (even though a slightly higher percentage may come from carbohydrates than fats), you are almost always using (burning) more total fat than if you worked at a lower intensity.

### Is it true you cannot be fit and fat at the same time?

Myth! You *can* be fit and fat. You can also be unfit and lean. Neither is ideal, however. Obesity and sedentary lifestyles independently accelerate arterial and immune aging, meaning heart disease, stroke, memory loss, impotence, wrinkles, infections, and cancer, not to mention arthritis and bone breaks and disability and pain. This means that you don't want to be either unfit or obese. If you are overweight and active, you reduce the risk of becoming big enough to be called "Refrigerator." You also reduce blood pressure and bad fats in your blood, increase good fats, and reduce the risk of breast cancer, prostate cancer, and colon cancer—all with physical activity.

### What about the no-pain-no-gain mantra?

Another myth. The brief answer is that if it hurts, stop. If you dread your workout, change it. The pursuit of a younger RealAge and fitness should be a joy and pleasure.

The longer answer is that most people realize—at least in an intellectual way—

that you do not need to put yourself through agony to reap health benefits. Walking in short bouts throughout the day is almost as beneficial as engaging in one longer walking session. And engaging in short bursts of high-intensity activity between periods of moderate-intensity activity provides as much benefit as working long and hard at a continuous high intensity.

So if that's true, why do so many people continue to abuse themselves with painful or unnecessarily long or grueling workouts? Why do more than thirty thousand people participate in the Chicago Marathon each year? Why are ultra-marathons becoming more popular? The answer is complicated, but here's a start: No truly educated people are doing these things for their health, whatever they say. There are probably more health-related reasons *not* to run a marathon than to run one. But completing something so physically challenging, for whatever reasons, brings certain psychological benefits. And we certainly do not dismiss such benefits.

If you are planning to enter a grueling event, make sure the emotional payoff is worth the physical and time sacrifices. You are not making yourself younger with the physical activity. Arnold said it best—he knows of no professional athlete who has not ruined their body for their sport. Yet we have talked with athletes who claimed that the satisfaction of engaging in their particular activity was well worth the arthritic shoulder or knee. Know the activity's risk and assess the perceived benefits you might gain from participation, and know that extreme physical activity isn't making your RealAge younger.

### Should exercise be painless?

Painless, yes (arthritis sufferers may be an exception), but not effortless. On the opposite side of the no-pain-no-gain camp lies the work-light-live-right camp. The work-light group rides the escalator rather than walks up the stairs. When asked about their exercise habits they often say, "I don't exercise, but I am very physically active." And they follow with a list of things they do, such as taking the dog for a walk, going shopping, and shuttling the kids here and there—activities that do not elevate their heart rates to a level 6 or 7 in intensity. These are not lazy people. They are active people, in a sense. But they are also not reaping the rewards that you will get from the RealAge Workout.

**I've heard that coenzyme (Co)Q10 will make me a better athlete. Is this true?**

This may be a myth. CoQ10 (aka ubiquinone) is an essential part of your cells that facilitates energy conversion (it helps convert glucose to ATP, which your muscles and other cells use). In a few studies, CoQ10 improved performance by 10 to 30 percent. But these benefits have not been replicated by most other studies. CoQ10 is a benefit if you are diabetic, hypertensive, have Parkinson's disease, or take a statin drug.

**How long will it take to get fit?**

That depends on what you do and how often, hard, and long you do it—also on your genetic makeup and your definition of the word *fit.*

Your body begins to reshape with your very first session and continues to adapt. In general, the adaptations occur more quickly and more dramatically the more often and the more intensely you work out. The most observable changes occur in the first few months of training.

Strength gains due to resistance training occur rapidly. During the first 8 to 10 weeks of training, the gains are largely attributable to neural factors, such as the ability to activate more muscle fibers to assist in overcoming resistance. After 10 weeks of training, most additional strength gain is due to an increase in the muscle's size. With a moderate-to-intense resistance-training program, most adults can expect to see a 25 percent to over a 100 percent increase in strength within 6 months of training.

No one can tell you exactly how long it will take you to get *fit.* But with the well-balanced stamina- and strength-building RealAge Workout program, you should notice improvements in your fitness within 4 to 6 weeks and likely even sooner. And if you are a 50-year-old woman with only 10 to 15 more pounds but less shape than you had at age 18, you can have that 18-year-old body doing the RealAge Workout in 2 to 3 years, and feel about 18 as well (but won't have to worry about acne). If you are concerned with quantifying your gains, fill out workout logs to document your progress.

**I'm an overweight exerciser and I chafe between my thighs—what can I do?**

This is a common question from large individuals who want to reduce weight. You can minimize the problem by wearing form-fitting clothes made from synthetic fibers like Lycra that wick away sweat. Dry all areas well, and dry again after cooling down in a half hour (use the bathroom to be discreet if you exercise or walk in the middle of the day, but do dry even if all you do is walk).

**Can my 16-year-old do the RealAge Workout with me?**

*(Weak data on this issue, so this is a best-guess answer.)* Yes, with you—but not for you. No substitutions, please. His or her exercising does not replace yours. (Soccer Moms and Dads please note: Pacing the sidelines instead of sitting in a chair are to be encouraged—the soccer field is a great place to motivate yourself with a pedometer to see if you can get younger while watching your children be active.) And no averaging, please. A 22,000-step day yesterday or a 60-minute walk yesterday does not replace 10,000 steps or 30 minutes today and every day.

Now, as to the 16-year-old working out with you, by all means do it, but make sure you vary the workout, especially if you are going to include a child below age 13. A 16-year-old can and should learn to weight-lift and do resistance exercises (girls as well as boys). Repetition is tough on young joints and especially the growth plates of bones—the part of the bone that is the weakest part of a child's bone structure because it hasn't calcified fully. So cross-train: treadmill one day, elliptical another, etc. And if your child is a daughter, remember to avoid twisting exercises in the peri-period time, as this is the time of most laxity of, and most twisting injuries to, her knee's anterior cruciate ligament.

**If I'm getting dehydrated, will I feel thirsty?**

You would think Mother Nature would have equipped us to feel thirsty immediately when we needed water. But she failed us. By the time your thirst mechanism kicks in and makes you want to drink, you are already mildly dehydrated. You will also stop feeling thirsty before you have drunk enough to become fully hydrated. In other words, relying on thirst to dictate your fluid intake will leave you in a constant state of mild dehydration. It's important to remain hydrated, so drink early and often, and remember to try a sports drink if you work out for more than an hour at a time.

**Can I exercise if I have arthritis?**

Yes. If you let arthritis keep you from moving, you will eventually lose your ability to move. People with arthritis often avoid moving a certain joint because the movement causes pain. Wrong, unfortunately! Neglecting the movement of a painful arthritic joint leads to increased stiffness and sometimes a shortening of the surrounding muscle and connective tissue, limiting the amount of possible movement at that joint. Limited movement means loss of mobility and function. To avoid this, keep moving.

Osteoarthritis is the most common form of arthritis—and sad but true, 95 percent of us will have osteoarthritis (according to X-ray) by the time calendar age 85 rolls around. X-ray abnormalities do not always mean the joint is painful, and painful joints do not always show X-ray abnormalities. But many people with arthritis have pain. Thus, people who have arthritis may be less likely to exercise, and for an obvious reason: It hurts. However, modest exercise (walking or swimming combined with lunges and squats) can actually *relieve* the symptoms of many types of arthritis. Furthermore, not exercising may cause the sudden appearance of arterial disease that could have been staved off with exercise.

The response to one chronic illness (say, a lack of walking due to arthritis) may bring about another chronic illness (arterial disease). But data from many well-known studies show that osteoarthritis progression can be stopped. A combination of calcium (600 mg twice a day), vitamin C (500 mg twice a day), vitamin D (200 IU twice a day), aspirin (162 mg a day with half a glass of warm water before and after), and exercise retarded the progression of osteoarthritis, and in some cases actually even prevented it. (Take only 100 mg of vitamin C if you are taking a statin drug for cholesterol management, as vitamins C and E interfere with the anti-inflammatory benefits of statins.)

Scientists and nutritionists have recently added another three agents—the first two are glucosamine and chondroitin—to the anti-arthritis arsenal. Glucosamine is a form of amino sugar that researchers believe plays a role in cartilage formation; chondroitin sulfate is part of the protein molecule that gives cartilage its elasticity. Taken in combination, the two do a good job of lessening the pain that often comes with arthritis. While there is recent controversy about this benefit, the preponderance of evidence favors a benefit.

But glucosamine and chondroitin do more than just treat pain. They also appear to be disease modifying, reversing some of the clinical and radiologic symptoms and evidence of joint disease. (For more info, go to www.drtheo.com, where Dr. Jason Theodosakis, an expert in this field, talks about the benefits of glucosamine and chondroitin sulfate, and lists the preparations he has tested that contain the necessary ingredients.)

The third agent that's been shown to reduce joint inflammation and delay or prevent arthritis is the omega-3 oils that are fish oils or DHA. To get these, take 2 gm of metabolically distilled fish oil daily (that's the kind on most shelves but look for the phrase "metabolically distilled" on the label) or the same amount of omega-3 fatty acids such as walnut oil or echium oil. Even simpler, just eat an ounce of walnuts a day, or fish (the typical 4-ounce serving) 3 times a week.

Osteoarthritis progresses slowly. If you manage it early and aggressively, you can continue to enjoy the activities you love—dancing, painting, gardening, whatever—without a whine or a whimper from those hips, knuckles, or knees. Remember your doctor doesn't take care of your body. That's your job, and a walk with stretches afterward is the best way to keep younger. The really good news, of course, is that doing the RealAge Workout activities actually helps prevent the aging that can come from arthritis.

### Should I weigh myself every morning?

Unless you are a truly quantitative person and need a running count of the pounds and ounces to keep you motivated, many would advise you to stop obsessing about weight. Concentrate instead on how good you feel when you exercise regularly.

But putting the scale in a closet may not be for everyone. Many successful weight controllers (people who have lost significant weight and kept it off for over 5 years) do indeed keep close track of their weight, but most usually keep detailed records of their eating and exercise habits as well. In studies of crash dieters who lost over 60 pounds in a short period of time and kept it off, more than 50 percent kept food and physical activity logs. That does not seem necessary for some who gradually lose weight, a situation that is much healthier.

I once had a client whose hourly moods seemed governed by what her scale told her. She weighed herself 3 or 4 times a day and would get depressed if her weight went up by a quarter pound between weigh-ins. I challenged her to go for a week without weighing herself. That was harder for her than quitting smoking. At the end of the week, she weighed in and found that she was half a pound less than the week before.

We gradually extended the time between weight checks to one month. The scale continued to show slow but consistent weight loss. Her best guess as to why she couldn't lose weight when she was checking it all the time was that her obsession about the weight constantly reminded her of food and feeling deprived. She ate more because food was brought to her attention so often. When she stopped dwelling on her weight, she stopped dwelling on food as well.

Conversely, I have another client who uses daily weight checks to his advantage. Not only do the weight checks help him alter his eating habits, the weight checks have also taught him much about the way his body responds to different foods. He can tell you which foods make him retain water and raise his blood pressure and/or his weight, the foods that make him feel like eating more and lead to weight gain, and the foods that satisfy him and lead to weight loss. He never lets his weight fluctuate by more than 3 pounds before making changes to bring his weight back where he wants it.

Wherever you stand on the issue, weigh yourself and measure your waist at least once a month (or once every 3 months as part of a quarterly assessment), and use the information for what it is—an indication of your weight and RealAge. A scale will not tell you how much of your weight is attributed to bone, fat, cartilage, or muscle. If you use the information in conjunction with other assessment tools such as waist circumference, it can help you evaluate the effects of your particular physical activity program. I am a big believer in waist measurements being the key measurement for this concern, and a tape measure being a key item in your bathroom or dressing area to assess your RealAge Workout progress.

### I'm an older person. How does physical exercise benefit me?

Physical exercise benefits the older person dramatically. As you age, your arteries become stiffer, so they cannot dilate as much. That dilation is what delivers nutrients to your bones and muscles, oxygen to your heart and increases your body's ability to remove toxins from your muscles. The 9- to 12-year-old can run all day because her arteries can dilate. But the 60-year-old feels tired chasing her grandchild because the 60-year-old's arteries are harder and not able to dilate as much. Physical activity—all three forms of it—enable your arteries to dilate and, in so doing, give you more energy.

At the same time, as you age, your muscle mass would decrease if you did nothing to make your RealAge younger by engaging in some form of strength training. Resistance (strength building) training thus makes you a fat-burning "trim" factory as opposed to a fat-storing "sack."

The benefits of physical activity for the older person do not stop here. Because of declines in the neuromuscular system that accompany chronological aging, your flexibility, balance, coordination, and reaction times decrease, inhibiting optimal function and increasing the risk of falls, accidents, and injury. These conditions make your RealAge older and impact your quality of life. Exercise maximizes the efficiency of the neuromuscular system, minimizing declines in flexibility, balance, and reaction times.

The importance of exercise for older people was demonstrated recently by a Canadian study of 98 women, 75 to 85 years old, all suffering from reduced bone mass or full-blown osteoporosis. After 6 months of exercising, those who engaged in 50-minute, twice-a-week strength training lowered their risk of falling by 57 percent.

Your older years can be your best years. This is something many of our patients tell us as soon as they've done physical activity for 90 days. Just enjoy adopting the workout as it is outlined in this book, while taking care to listen to your body and not pushing yourself too hard when you don't feel up to it.

If you cannot sustain a physical activity such as walking for 30 consecutive minutes, divide your 30 minutes of exercise into two or more shorter, nonconsecutive sessions. For instance, you might try three separate 10-minute sessions. Your RealAge will be just as young. If you keep this up, over time your endurance will almost certainly improve, enabling you eventually to accomplish a 30-minute workout. If, however, you cannot increase your duration beyond 10 minutes, don't be discouraged. Several short bouts of exercise each day go a long, long way.

There are two important things for the older person to remember during a workout. First, the older body may require a little more time to adapt to the stresses of an exercise session, so be sure to allow 5 to 10 minutes for your warm-up. Second, as you age, your sensation of thirst diminishes. Even younger people can become dehydrated before they feel thirsty. Force yourself to take frequent water breaks.

■　　■　　■

So one final wish for all who have made it this far: May you find a RealAge walking and workout partner and enjoy getting younger together. And remember to celebrate with year-younger birthday parties. There is no reason not to postpone disability and increase your quality of life every year. The RealAge Workout is too easy.

# Appendix

## Reliable Internet Sources for Fitness Information

### 1. American College of Sports Medicine (www.acsm.org)

The American College of Sports Medicine has developed a series of "Current Comments" available to the general public. Go to the website, scroll down the left side to "Public Resources," and then click "Current Comments." The comments contain accurate information on a variety of topics (almost 50 comments are currently online), including exercise and age-related weight gain, overtraining, exercise during pregnancy, tennis elbow, and vitamin and mineral supplements.

### 2. American Council on Exercise (www.acefitness.org)

The ACE website is extremely accessible and helpful for finding reliable fitness information on interesting and frequently thought-about topics. Click on "ACE Fit Facts" to find almost 100 easy-to-understand articles in 12 different categories.

**3. Our websites (www.RealAgeWorkout.com, www.RealAge.com and www.youtheownersmanual.com)**

We don't mean to brag, but we reference and run all data we post by a panel of experts. Enjoy the websites—they're there for you!

## Rules for Everyone

Every journey begins with a single step. Here's the one I want you to take. Here is a page containing the RealAge Workout rules. Xerox it and stick it on your fridge, your front door, a mirror, whatever—just so long as it's in a place you go to many times during the day.

Your job—your first step on the RealAge journey to making yourself feel, look, and act younger—is to read the rules every chance you get. Study them. Think about them often, when you're awake and when you're sleeping. And above all, do them.

### The RealAge Workout Rules

1. Commit to and start a program of physical activity—and do it today.
2. Walk first.
3. Engage in some physical activity every day.
4. Do not increase your physical activity by more than 10 percent any week, no matter how good you feel.
5. A watch is your key piece of equipment.
6. Exercise should not be painful. Stop if it hurts.
7. Warm up before you start and always stretch when you're done.
8. Prevent joint and muscle inflammation by taking an aspirin or a non-steroidal anti-inflammatory drug 2 hours before you begin your physical activity, if your doctor agrees.
9. Drink *before* you get thirsty.
10. When increasing stamina activity, push yourself to an uncomfortable or just barely comfortable level for at least 30 seconds every 7 minutes.
11. Cross-train.

12. Reward yourself. Set goals and treat yourself—celebrate—when you achieve those goals.

13. For a double benefit of friendship and stress relief, exercise with a friend.

14. Take a lesson: Even if you don't normally work out with a trainer or a pro, she can show you how to maximize your workout and avoid needless injuries.

15. Vary your workout pace. Do more on some days and less on others.

16. Strengthen your 7 foundation muscle groups first.

17. Never sacrifice form for added weight.

18. Train at threshold—use a weight you can lift properly only 8 to 12 times before your muscle fully fatigues.

19. Do not take a weight past 90 degrees of joint movement for any one exercise unless I say to do so.

20. Breathe when lifting.

## Crib Sheets (feel free to Xerox for yourself)

*A Crib Sheet on the Physical Activity That Will Make Your RealAge the Youngest It Can Be*

| WHEN TO START | WHAT TO START | HOW MUCH TO DO AT FIRST |
|---|---|---|
| Day 1 | Walking | No more than 3 minutes more than you do usually. How fast: only as fast as you are comfortable |
| Day 1 | Stretches for walking | 2 minutes a day |
| Day 31 | Resistance exercises for foundation muscles | 7 minutes every even-numbered day |
| Day 31 | Stretches for foundation muscles | 1–2 minutes every even-numbered day |
| Day 61 | Resistance exercises for non-foundation muscles | 6 minutes every even-numbered day* |
| Day 61 | Stretches for non-foundation muscles | 1–2 minutes every even-numbered day |
| Day 91 | Stamina activity | As much as you usually do, or start with 8 minutes with at least 1 minute at threshold (as much as you can do†) on odd or even days |
| Day 91 | Stretches for stamina exercises | 2 minutes every day you do stamina—you can combine with other stretches if you do resistance or walking at the same time |

* Can be done on every odd or every even numbered day—one or the other, not switching back and forth—whatever suits your schedule.
† If you are over age 33, do only after an okay from your physician, or if you are already doing these exercises.

| HOW MUCH TO BUILD TO PER WEEK | WHEN TO END | WHERE TO FIND HOW TO DO IN THIS BOOK |
|---|---|---|
| Build by increasing no more than 5 minutes per day every week until you hit 30 minutes a day | Never—if it rains, walk; if it snows, walk; if there's a hurricane, or an earthquake—walk, or better yet, run | Chapters 1 and 2 |
| 2 minutes a day | Never | Chapter 2 |
| 7 minutes every even-numbered day—increase dumbbell or machine weight no more than 10% in any week | Never—if you injure a key muscle group, do this activity using uninjured muscles | Chapter 3 |
| 2 minutes every even-numbered day | Never | Chapter 2 |
| 8 minutes every even-numbered day—increase dumbbell or machine weight no more than 10% any week | Never—if you injure a key muscle group, do this activity using uninjured muscles | Chapter 4 |
| 2 minutes every even-numbered day | Never | Chapters 2 and 4 |
| 21 minutes 3 times a week of sweating activity or at 80% of maximum heart rate, with at least 1 minute every 7 at threshold (maximum you can do). Increase no more than 10% any week | If you have a viral infection, decrease activity; if you injure a key muscle group, do this activity using uninjured muscles | Chapter 5 |
| 2 minutes every day you do stamina activity | Never | Chapter 5 |

# Suggested First 120-Day RealAge Workout Plan and More

| DAY | PHYSICAL ACTIVITY | PLANNING ACTIVITY (OR PHYSICAL ACTIVITY) |
|---|---|---|
| | | (You can vary the day you do any of these activities planned for the first 11 days to fit into your available time, but I suggest you do all of these activities within the first 11 days.) |
| 1 | ☐ Walk 30 min | ☐ Read Chapters 1 and 2 |
| 2 | ☐ Walk 30 min ☐ Do stretches | ☐ Read Chapter 3 |
| | | ☐ Do Assessment (pages 24–25) |
| 3 | ☐ Walk 30 min ☐ Do stretches | ☐ Read Chapter 4 ☐ Throw out "white food"* |
| 4 | ☐ Walk 30 min ☐ Do stretches | ☐ Repopulate your kitchen with healthy food |
| 5 | ☐ Walk 30 min ☐ Do stretches | ☐ Investigate and buy new walking/workout shoes |
| 6 | ☐ Walk 30 min ☐ Do stretches | ☐ Investigate health clubs/gyms/trainers nearby |
| 7 | ☐ Walk 30 min ☐ Do stretches | ☐ Read Chapter 5 |
| 8 | ☐ Walk 30 min ☐ Do stretches | ☐ Read Chapter 6 |
| 9 | ☐ Walk 30 min ☐ Do stretches | ☐ Schedule trainer appointments for days 31/33/37, 61/63 |
| 10 | ☐ Walk 30 min ☐ Do stretches | ☐ Schedule physician appointments for day 30 or 60 |
| 11 | ☐ Walk 30 min ☐ Do stretches | ☐ Reinvigorate your kitchen with fruits/ veggies, balsalmic vinegar, and healthy fats* |
| 12–16 | ☐ Walk 30 min ☐ Do stretches | |
| 17 | ☐ Walk 30 min ☐ Do stretches | ☐ Reinvigorate your kitchen with fruits/veggies* |
| 18–22 | ☐ Walk 30 min ☐ Do stretches | |
| 23 | ☐ Walk 30 min ☐ Do stretches | ☐ Reinvigorate your kitchen with fruits/veggies* |
| 24–28 | ☐ Walk 30 min ☐ Do stretches | |
| 29 | ☐ Walk 30 min ☐ Do stretches | ☐ Reinvigorate your kitchen with fruits/veggies* |
| 30 | ☐ Walk 30 min ☐ Do stretches | ☐ See physician—discuss your physical activity plan |
| 31 | ☐ Walk 30 min ☐ Do stretches | ☐ 1st training session for foundation exercises |
| 32 | ☐ Walk 30 min ☐ Do stretches | |
| 33 | ☐ Walk 30 min ☐ Do stretches | ☐ 2nd training session for foundation exercises |
| 34 | ☐ Walk 30 min ☐ Do stretches | ☐ Reinvigorate your kitchen with fruits/ veggies* |
| 35 | ☐ Walk 30 min ☐ Do stretches | ☐ Foundation strengthening exercises on own |
| 36 | ☐ Walk 30 min ☐ Do stretches | |
| 37 | ☐ Walk 30 min ☐ Do stretches | ☐ Review session with trainer for foundation exercises |

* See *RealAge® Makeover* for more information.

| | | |
|---|---|---|
| 38 | ☐ Walk 30 min ☐ Do stretches | |
| 39 | ☐ Walk 30 min ☐ Do stretches | ☐ Foundation strengthening |
| 40 | ☐ Walk 30 min ☐ Do stretches | |
| 41 | ☐ Walk 30 min ☐ Do stretches | ☐ Foundation strengthening |
| 42 | ☐ Walk 30 min ☐ Do stretches | ☐ Reinvigorate your kitchen with fruits/veggies* |
| 43 | ☐ Walk 30 min ☐ Do stretches | ☐ Foundation strengthening |
| 44–60 | Repeat 38–43 in sequence | |
| 61 | ☐ Walk 30 min ☐ Do stretches | ☐ 1st training session for non-foundation exercises |
| 62 | ☐ Walk 30 min ☐ Do stretches | |
| 63 | ☐ Walk 30 min ☐ Do stretches | ☐ 2nd training session for non-foundation exercises |
| 64 | ☐ Walk 30 min ☐ Do stretches | ☐ Reinvigorate your kitchen with fruits/veggies* |
| 65 | ☐ Walk 30 min ☐ Do stretches | ☐ Foundation and non-foundation strengthening exercises on own |
| 66 | ☐ Walk 30 min ☐ Do stretches | |
| 67 | ☐ Walk 30 min ☐ 10 min strengthening exercises | ☐ Do stretches |
| 68 | ☐ Walk 30 min ☐ Do stretches | |
| 69 | ☐ Walk 30 min ☐ 10 mins strengthening exercises | ☐ Do stretches |
| 70 | ☐ Walk 30 min ☐ Do stretches | ☐ Reinvigorate your kitchen with fruits/veggies* |
| 71–89 | Repeat 66–70 in sequence | |
| 90 | ☐ Walk 30 min ☐ Do repeat assessment | ☐ Do stretches |
| 91 | ☐ Walk 30 min ☐ Do stretches | ☐ Review session for strengthening exercises |
| 92 | ☐ Walk 30 min ☐ Find stamina exercise you like for 21 min | ☐ Do stretches |
| 93 | ☐ Walk 30 min ☐ 10 min strengthening exercises | ☐ Do stretches |
| 94 | ☐ Walk 30 min ☐ Stamina exercise you like for 21 min | ☐ Do stretches |
| 95 | ☐ Walk 30 min ☐ Do stretches | ☐ Reinvigorate your kitchen with fruits/veggies* |
| 96 | ☐ Walk 30 min ☐ Stamina exercise you like for 21 min | ☐ Do stretches |
| 97 | ☐ Walk 30 min ☐ 10 min strengthening exercises | ☐ Do stretches |
| 98–119 | Repeat sequence of numbers 92–97 | |
| 120 | ☐ Walk 30 min ☐ Do repeat assessment | ☐ Do stretches |

* See *RealAge® Makeover* for more information.

# Index

# About the Authors

## About Michael F. Roizen, M.D.

Dr. Roizen is a professor of internal medicine and anesthesiology and chair of the Division of Anesthesiology, Critical Care Medicine, and Comprehensive Pain Management at the Cleveland Clinic. He developed the RealAge® program while trying to motivate patients to lower their risk of complications of surgery by adopting healthier lifestyles. Dr. Roizen is a Phi Beta Kappa graduate of Williams College and Alpha Omega Alpha graduate of the University of California, San Francisco, Medical School. He is 60 calendar years of age, but his RealAge is 42.1.

Dr. Roizen is past chair of a Food and Drug Administration advisory committee; has been an editor for six medical journals; and has published more than 155 peer-reviewed scientific papers, 100 textbook chapters, 30 editorials, and four medical books. Dr. Roizen is the founder of RealAge, Inc., a San Diego–based company, which includes an interactive Web site located at www.RealAge.com. The site addresses health and wellness issues, and the RealAge "Tip of the Day" is subscribed to by more than 4.4 million people in North America. Dr. Roizen has also developed a program first launched at Northwestern Memorial Hospital aimed at helping its members to become smart patients and reverse biologic aging and live longer, more vibrant lives.

Dr. Roizen's first book, *RealAge®: Are You As Young As You Can Be?* hit #1 on the *New York Times* list, and other successful books include *The RealAge® Makeover* and two books written with Dr. John La Puma, *Cooking the RealAge® Way,* and *The RealAge® Diet,* which was also a *New York Times* best seller. Dr. Roizen's most recent book, *YOU: The Owner's Manual,* cowritten with Dr. Mehmet C. Oz, was also a blockbuster best seller, hitting #1 on the *New York Times* list.

Dr. Roizen's wife is a developmental pediatrician. They have two children—Jenny, a Ph.D. graduate student at Caltech in organic chemistry, and Jeffrey, an M.D./Ph.D. student at Washington University in St Louis.

## About Tracy Hafen, M.S.

Tracy Hafen is the head of Exercise Physiology at the Center for Partnership Medicine at Northwestern Memorial Hospital. Tracy has a master's degree in exercise science and cardiac rehabilitation, and she graduated from Brigham Young University.

In 1994, Tracy cofounded Affirmative Fitness, one of Chicago's premiere personal fitness training companies. In Tracy's work with private clients, she has focused on strength-training programs, sports training, weight management, and general fitness. Tracy and her husband, Tom, have six children.